AS REAL AS IT GETS

AS REAL AS IT GETS

The Life of a Hospital at the Center of the AIDS Epidemic

Carol Pogash

Foreword by
Randy Shilts

A BIRCH LANE PRESS BOOK
Published by Carol Publishing Group

A Birch Lane Press Book
Published by Carol Publishing Group
Birch Lane Press is a registered trademark of Carol Communications, Inc.
Editorial Offices: 600 Madison Avenue, New York, N.Y. 10022
Sales and Distribution Offices: 120 Enterprise Avenue, Secaucus,
    N.J. 07094
In Canada: Canadian Manda Group, P.O. Box 920, Station U, Toronto,
    Ontario M8Z 5P9
Queries regarding rights and permissions should be addressed to
Carol Publishing Group, 600 Madison Avenue, New York, N.Y. 10022

Carol Publishing Group books are available at special discounts for
bulk purchases, for sales promotion, fund-raising, or educational
purposes. Special editions can be created to specifications. For
details, contact: Special Sales Department, Carol Publishing
Group, 120 Enterprise Avenue, Secaucus, N.J. 07094

Manufactured in the United States of America
10 9 8 7 6 5 4 3 2 1

Library of Congress Cataloging-in-Publication Data
Pogash, Carol.
    As real as it gets : the life of a hospital at the center of the
AIDS epidemic / Carol Pogash ; foreword by Randy Shilts.
        p.   cm.
    "A Birch Lane Press book."
    Includes index.
    ISBN 1-55972-127-8
        1. AIDS (Disease)   2. San Francisco General Hospital (Calif.)
    I. Title.
    RC607.A26P63   1992
    362.1'9697'9200979461—dc20   92-28516
                                                             CIP

To the nurses and doctors
at San Francisco General Hospital and
especially to Jane Doe,
for her spirit, humor
and willingness to tell her story.

Contents

Foreword

Nestled among the hills on the eastern edge of San Francisco, beside a freeway, is a cluster of red-brick and gray-concrete buildings that is the epicenter of the AIDS epidemic in America. From the epidemic's first mysterious days in 1981, every conflict, controversy and human drama inherent in the spread of a deadly new disease has been played out in that cluster of buildings called San Francisco General Hospital.

It is a truism of journalism that the stories that tell the larger tales often have the tighter focus. By focusing solely on the travails of just this one hospital in her book *As Real As It Gets*, Carol Pogash has artfully told the larger story of the AIDS epidemic. Anyone who reads a newspaper in San Francisco knows Carol as one of California's most incisive and lucid journalists. This book reflects her reportorial skill and reveals her also to be a gifted writer, able to weave the woof of human lives to the warp of history.

The importance of San Francisco General Hospital in the history of the AIDS epidemic cannot be overstated. The model of care now used the world over was pioneered in those buildings; the drugs used to treat hundreds of thousands of HIV patients were first tested there; the political controversies that would later ignite protesters nationwide were born there. The story of San Francisco General Hospital and the HIV pandemic provides a litany of firsts: General was the first hospital to have an inpatient HIV ward, the first to have an outpatient HIV clinic, the first institution outside the federal government to investigate the sexual behavior that might spread the disease, and the first to realize that the old way that hospitals cared for their patients needed to be changed if the institution was going to be able to cope with this horrible new disease.

The accumulation of superlatives for its AIDS care put San Francisco General in circumstances that it, or few other public hospitals for that matter, had ever confronted. While patients would once have done anything to avoid care in the county hospital, they were now clamoring to be admitted there. As the treatment became more skillful, august medical experts from around the world crowded the halls, too, to see how it was done. The doctors from San Francisco General became the international authorities on AIDS care. Situated in the city with the highest concentration of AIDS patients in the Western world, the hospital found itself constantly breaking new ground on the complicated medical, social, ethical and political issues that the epidemic animated.

These issues are the grist of *As Real As It Gets*, but this is no dry dissertation. This book's unique ability not only to explain ideas but to explore the human dimensions of the epidemic is what makes it such a valuable contribution to AIDS literature, as well as such a good read. We learn not only about what it takes to provide good AIDS care, but the life stories of the doctors and nurses and patients who were first challenged with how to develop care models and explore their fears and frustrations. The specifics of their jobs may have been unique to AIDS, but their ethical dilemmas and anxieties speak to issues touching all of society.

This truth is probably no more evident than in the sections of the book exploring the development of drugs to treat AIDS, particularly the bitter controversy over Compound Q, a treatment first developed and tested at San Francisco General. Here, the stories of AIDS activists and laboratory researchers and exasperated patients collide amid angry accusations and the ever-pressing deadlines imposed by the relentless human immunodeficiency virus. It's tough to pick out the good guys and bad guys, and Carol doesn't try to oversimplify the moral quandaries by doing that.

By telling the larger story of AIDS through the lives that people the halls of this one hospital, Pogash brings to life a compelling cast of characters. Take handsome young Dr. Michael McGrath, the dedicated laboratory researcher who develops an AIDS drug that, he expects, will make him a hero, though he is later accused of being a "murderer." There are the compassionate young doctors like Paul Volberding, Donald Abrams and Constance Wofsy, who see their careers hijacked by a disease none could have imagined just a few years earlier in their medical schools. They become medical celebrities while braving some of the most dispiriting work of any modern medical professionals. There are the dissenters, such as Dr. Lorraine Day, the attractive surgeon who becomes a star of the television talk-show circuit because of her factious calls for the AIDS testing of all her scheduled surgical patients. And there is the poignant story of Jane Doe, the idealistic twenty-four-year-old nurse who contracts HIV from a needle-stick and then does prolonged battle with a heartless city bureaucracy to receive her disability compensation.

As Real As It Gets also records the insidious spread of the epidemic out of the gay community and into the underclass, the impoverished inner-city youths, the despairing drug addicts and the prostitutes who are making up a larger share of this public hospital's caseload. Like many hospitals across the country, HIV-positive patients at General are no longer confined to the AIDS ward. One-quarter of those seeking services at the hospital are now thought to be AIDS infected, and their stories are recounted here as well.

There is not a drama inherent to the AIDS epidemic that has not been acted out in San Francisco General Hospital, whether over arguments of AIDS care or AIDS drugs or patient testing or health-care-worker risk. All these stories can be found on the pages that follow. *As Real As It Gets* is less a journalistic account than a parable of AIDS in America today. Right until the book's chilling last moment, the stories reveal that sometimes we have behaved well in the face of AIDS, and sometimes we have behaved poorly, and always we have behaved as humans, for better and for worse.

I first went to cover AIDS at San Francisco General Hospital in October 1983, just three months after it opened the world's first "AIDS ward." The patients were brave and talked optimistically about how they were going to stick it out, because they wanted to be around for the cure that must be just around the corner. The nurses were a proud and team-spirited group, eager to show the world that there were other ways to deal with AIDS than through hysteria. One evening for a Halloween party, a local cabaret singer named Sharon McKnight came to the ward in her sequined black gown and a long feathered boa, and entertained the patients with her trademark song, "Stand By Your Man." It was a festive and happy occasion.

I did not then know anyone who had died of AIDS, though a handful of acquaintances were sick, so, like everyone else, I had this can-do attitude toward the disease. We could provide the best treatment, keep people alive, the cure would come, and then we would have another party to celebrate the end of AIDS. Sharon McKnight could sing then, too; maybe some of the patients would still be alive to join in the revelry; the nightmare would be behind us.

That was nearly a decade ago. All the patients I interviewed for that first story are long since dead. As for myself, I once kept a mental list of all the friends who had died, but when one friend died last Sunday, one week to the day after another had died, I realized that I no longer kept any sort of tally. It was better to think of them one corpse at a time; taken together, the totality of death was too much to ponder. It was not the way to adapt.

Now the AIDS wards are not just at General but at hospitals through-out San Francisco. All the grim projections of future deaths that I reported in 1983 and 1984 have come true. Nurses talk about surviving grief overload and job burnout, not merely allaying hysteria. Though scientific advances are being made toward treatments, no one fantasizes plans for the day when the cure is found. One's aspiration is not to be at some AIDS-ending festival in the years ahead; the goal is to keep sane today and tomorrow and perhaps the next day and not become over-whelmed by the burden of death and despair. The story I wrote from those first days of the AIDS ward in 1983 was as grim as anything I had ever composed in my career to that point. Today, the memories seem almost ebullient and lighthearted compared to the reality that has unfolded in the decade since.

Someday, the AIDS epidemic will be over. The AIDS ward will shut down; the AIDS clinic will see its last patient. And we will sing and celebrate the end of the nightmare. When that day comes, *As Real As It Gets* will still be an invaluable document, a record of all that was human in our response to this troubled time.

—Randy Shilts
Guerneville, California

Acknowledgments

Dozens of people helped me write the book. This list could never be more than partial. I'd especially like to thank my main characters for sharing their lives with me: Nurse Jane Doe; Dr. Paul Volberding; Dr. Molly Cooke; Dr. Bill Schecter; Dr. John Luce; Dr. Lorraine Day; Gary Carr, RN, MS; Marley Gevanthor, RN; J.B. Molaghan, RN, ANP; Vince DeGenova, RN; Cliff Morrison, RN, FAAN; Dr. Michael McGrath; Dr. Gerald Hill; Dr. Melissa Bartick; Dr. Eric Goosby; Andrew Moss, Ph.D.; Judith Cohen, Ph.D.; Mary Rathbun.

Other people at the General and elsewhere who helped me include Dr. Donald Abrams; former San Francisco mayor Art Agnos; Dr. Constance Wofsy; Isabelle Gaston; Chris Adams; Carol Adams; Terry Beswick; Larry Bush; Fay Champoux; Andrea Crawford; Lenore Chinn; Joe Cowan; Diane Cirincione; Martin Delaney; Dr. Selma Dritz; Dr. Dick Fine; Rita Fahrner, RN; Carol Fink, RN; Carol Fox; Gayling Gee, RN, MS; Jayne Garrison; Wiley Herring; Patricia Hastings; Elaine Herscher; Vince Huang; Janet Pomeroy; Sue Kiely, RN; Dr. Jim Kahn;

Penni Kimmell; Dr. Gifford Leoung; Rabbi Pinchas Lipner; Tony Lobb, RN; Dr. Michon Morita; Clare Murphy; Toni Maines, RN; Alise Martinez, RN; Marti Nash, RN; Norm Nickens; Rose Pak; Dr. Herbert Perkins; Michelle Roland; Cathy Roseberry; Dr. Merle Sande; Jean Smith, RN; Phillip Sowa; Dr. Mervyn Silverman; Black Star; the late Dan Turner; Allan Temko; Dr. Mark Tonelli and many others. Despite their crammed schedules, everyone I talked to sat down for lengthy taped interviews and then let me follow them around.

Throughout the book I have substituted pseudonyms for the names of patients and of Jane Doe's friends. I appreciate their willingness to let me listen and observe.

I also must thank the federal Centers for Disease Control for their readiness to answer all my questions. I can't imagine writing a serious piece without the help of the librarians at the Berkeley Public Library's reference desk. Without them, I could not function.

Some of the General's top physicians and nurses working in AIDS are not in this book. I am only sorry I could not tell everyone's story. To those of you not in it, I apologize.

Since you never know how many times you have a chance to thank the people, I'd also add to this list my parents, Sylvia and Israel Pogash, for teaching me the importance of hard work, honesty, never taking no for an answer, and plain sentences. To my sister, Susan Pogash, who is always there for me and to my brother-in-law, Dr. Richard Karrel, for answering all my stupid questions and never laughing. And to my cousin, Dr. Henry Krumholz, for his help.

I am grateful to my husband, Jim Wood, editor of my words and life, for encouraging me when almost no one else did and for making his sensational dinners every night. Our children, Jacob and Rachel, have missed numerous chemistry experiments and visits to the park tire swing, respectively, while their mother was obsessively at work. My wonderful stepson, John Wood, and our family friend Stacy Lauer helped with the younger kids while I was downstairs tapping away at the computer.

Thank you to my editor, Bruce Shostak, who did a fine job under terrific time pressure. My agents Helen Meyer and Michaela Clavell were dedicated to selling my book even when they were warned that books on AIDS don't sell. Without their zeal and their contacts, this book would not have seen print. And to Randy Shilts, reporter extraordinaire, for willing this book into publication.

In the mid-eighties, employees in the hospital's emergency room sported a T-shirt reading *We Beat the Grim Reaper*. In the era of AIDS, it no longer seemed accurate. The new T-shirt read *This Is As Real As It Gets*.

SPRING AND SUMMER
1987

The Mistake

Every workday that spring and early summer she bounded up the concrete steps, across the parklike setting trimmed with pink and rose impatiens and white alyssum, past the slow gait of the tired, the sickly and the homeless, through the sterile glass doors of San Francisco General Hospital. At twenty-four, nursing was her calling, especially nursing at the county hospital.

She'd tried the role of subservient nurse, inching tissue boxes closer to bedsides, accommodating rich patients at expensive hospitals. That wasn't her style. Here, patients were not just in need of care, they were desperately in need of it. When, as at the General, patients were at the cusp of death, she found that "the curtain of B.S. is completely cut away. Human beings are out there with their feelings."

She preferred working with the sickest of patients, including those with AIDS. Others might be afraid of them, afraid of contracting the disease. She felt invulnerable. Contracting AIDS from a patient, she

3

thought, was about as likely as being mowed down by a tractor. She didn't think about either one very often.

For several months she reveled in her new post, working twelve-hour shifts. Just after 6 A.M., on the last hour of her day on a cool July morning, the nurse erred. It was the kind of mistake that less experienced nurses make.

An AIDS patient had medicine infusing from a bag through IV tubing into a catheter (a little hollow plastic tube) that had been placed in his vein. The IV tubing was connected to a rubber port by a needle. When the medicine ran out, the tubing could be removed while the catheter remained in place. That way, the patient could avoid another puncture.

The patient's medicine had run out and his blood was backing up into his IV tubing. The nurse removed the IV tubing from the rubber port and stood at his bed with the unsheathed needle at the end of the rubber tubing.

She wasn't supposed to recap the needle. Hospital policy declared such moves too risky. Jostle a finger an eighth of an inch in the wrong direction and you could stick yourself. The joke around the hospital was that if you pricked yourself, play it safe: cut off your finger.

She was supposed to weave through the room with the metal pole, bag and unsheathed needle, like a player completing an obstacle course. She was going to have to maneuver her way to the bathroom to toss the used needle into the narrow-necked Sharps box, the discard receptacle. It would have made more sense for the shiny red Sharps box to be hinged on the wall by the patient's bed, but hospital administrators had insisted it be hidden from public view to dissuade passing drug addicts or the curious from wandering by to fish out needles.

The procedure seemed too hard and too risky. Instead, the nurse held the back of the IV bag steady, sticking the needle with the patient's blood into its rubber port.

Her right hand slipped. The needle pierced the IV bag, puncturing her left index finger. A deep stick. She squeezed her finger, bled it out. She scrubbed her hand and did what she was supposed to do. She told the charge nurse.

"Oh," said her sympathetic superior. "It's always hardest the first time."

THE BEGINNING
1981

The Crumbling Wall

No one predicted Dr. Paul Volberding would become a medical superstar: not his medical-school classmates or his fellow residents. Even in his marriage to the willowy Dr. Molly Cooke, she was the academically flashy mate. But behind the image—he resembled a young Marlon Brando—were the qualities patients seek in the finest physicians. And all the character that Volberding possessed was called into action in July 1981, when he began an oncology clinic at San Francisco General Hospital.

His was a pocket-size clinic. He had no grants, no cancer drug trials, no lab and no employees. And he had little reason to think he could financially sustain the work. He thought he was being set up to fail. In fact, he would never find out.

On Volberding's first day, he visited the bedside of a twenty-two-year-old southern man dying for no apparent reason. With mottled purple lesions, he was the General's first patient with Kaposi's sarcoma, a rare skin cancer known to afflict old Jewish, Greek, Italian and African men and believed to be relatively benign. The patient looked to be in his fifties or sixties with eyes so full of pain they were nearly lifeless. His body had wasted until he was a skeleton wrapped in skin. To Volberding, he resembled the prisoners in the black-and-white photos snapped at the liberation of Auschwitz. The patient's image would imprint on the physician's mind.

Other patients with the same disease trickled in. In time, a torrent of them would overflow the corridors and the city's medical system. At the epicenter of the epidemic, San Francisco General came to reflect all that was good and sometimes bad about the way doctors and nurses responded to the frightening disease. Volberding's reflexive response—to treat, to learn and to care—elevated his life and that of the General, making it the finest and most famous AIDS hospital in the world. But Volberding recognized none of that when he examined his patient.

The frail man with a southern accent had worked in the city's gay bathhouses, the ultimate in uncomplicated, impersonal gay sex. When Volberding and oncology fellow Ray Stricker examined him, they didn't have a clue what was going on. But Stricker recalled seeing patients like this one in New York City, where he had just completed his residency at Roosevelt Hospital. Stricker called his East Coast colleagues, but no one in New York seemed to know anything about the strange illness either. Four days later, the federal Centers for Disease Control reported on the first cases of KS in gay men in New York and California.

Volberding treated the patient for cancer because he didn't know what else to do. The illness was so rare the doctor had to scour medical libraries for information. The few articles he found said nothing about wasting nor about the opportunistic infections the doctors would later see in their patients.

With no friends or family, the patient reached out to his physician and to the clinic's nurse, Gayling Gee, hired that autumn. Sometimes he would wait outside the doorway of the clinic a half hour before it opened. Other times, Gee found him waiting inside, drinking a carton of milk, munching a cookie and complaining that he had no place to stay. Unprepared, Gee learned fast where to find resources for this patient and those who were to follow.

When the man developed a pneumonia that autumn, the doctors conducted an open-lung biopsy. While in the intensive care unit, recovering from the surgery, the patient died.

Earlier, patients with the mysterious, unidentified illness had come through the hospital. Dr. Constance Wofsy had seen a gay man thought to be suffering from a brain tumor and pneumonia. When she threw out the wild suggestion that his illness might have something to do with his being gay, everyone agreed there could be no relevance.

Internist Molly Cooke had seen a young gay man with toxoplasmosis, a parasitic disease found in cats and seen in immuno-suppressed people. The disease had infected the patient's brain. When Cooke sent slides to a renowned expert, he told her she must have made a mistake in her diagnosis because healthy people don't get toxoplasmosis.

No one yet had a sense that this was a worldwide epidemic unfolding in the white sheets of county hospital beds.

That fall, Volberding, a University of California Medical School assistant professor, bumped into Dr. Marcus Conant, a UCSF dermatologist. He learned that Conant, too, had seen a handful of KS patients. Together they examined a patient and began a collaboration between the bold, older physician, with established contacts in the gay community, and the less experienced but more diplomatic one—a partnership that would benefit their patients and the city of San Francisco. Under Conant's leadership, information was shared among physicians at the university, the General and in the city's health department. Regularly Conant and Volberding went to local gay political groups to tell them what they knew about the deadly "gay cancer," or what was called GRID for gay-related immune deficiency, even when they didn't know very much.

It didn't take more than ten cases for the doctors to realize they were observing an amazing illness they'd never seen before. Volberding found it "striking how incredibly complex, how multisystemic it was, how little we understood and how powerless we were to do anything." But the sadness of caring for dying men barely old enough to vote was balanced by the excitement Volberding felt every time he examined a new patient. The learning curve was so steep that doctors likened it to scaling a cliff. At the General, physicians saw the first case of cryptococcus, a virulent fungal infection; the first toxoplasmosis of the brain probably anywhere in the world. With Dr. Jerome Groopman, his counterpart at the University of California at Los Angeles School of Medicine, Volberding wrote a letter to the *New England Journal of Medicine* describing their first patients with Septra rashes (a blotchy, itchy red rash, it is an allergic reaction experienced by 60 percent of patients given Septra, a drug used to fight Pneumocystis carinii pneumonia), a reaction that became so common that a few years later, every medical student in the nation would know to look for it in AIDS patients.

It was impossible to see one of these patients and not come away very impressed by this illness.

Those involved from the beginning knew almost immediately that what they were doing was important. It made Volberding feel sorry for people who ask themselves at the end of each day, "Is what I'm doing worthwhile?" Volberding, however, asked himself, "Can I keep this up?"

Still, his work was not viewed as anything that could help his academic career. Volberding's colleagues did not consider GRID to be a real disease. Academically speaking, many felt it wasn't going to go anywhere. For Volberding to succeed at the University of California Medical School in San Francisco, or in academic medicine anywhere, he was supposed to find an area he could research and then publish his findings. And while GRID clearly was a big deal, it was not at all clear that it was going to be an academic big deal. But Volberding's patients pulled him in.

Other doctors, even many at the General, shied away from the GRID patients, which was why the inexperienced oncologist with almost no staff and no real status cared for them. Even at this tolerant county hospital, where an elevator ride can be a cross-cultural experience, many health-care workers were not pleased to have the men with the frightening disease flocking to their doors. At the same time, many at the General sighed a collective "thank God" that Volberding was willing to care for them. Sometimes he was asked by colleagues why he would want to specialize in "the homosexual disease." He'd respond, "It was fascinating to me from day one."

Volberding was born not so much a leader as he was an adapter. A buffeted middle child, he learned to compromise, mediate and sometimes play one side off against the other, skills that would help him build support for his program in the hospital and in the gay community.

He'd grown up on a Minnesota farm, raised championship Jerseys and been a member of the 4H Club, a cultural experience quite distinct from gay life in San Francisco. Living in Rochester, home of the Mayo Clinic, the young Volberding observed that the model of success was a doctor, although his family didn't always take the advice of the medical community. Despite the doctors' advice at the time, his parents chose not to institutionalize his brother Mark, who had Down's syndrome, caring for him at home instead. In ways that Volberding can't describe, having a brother like Mark made him more sensitive to the plight of others. And his parents' willingness to oppose the medical establishment gave the doctor a model of personal courage that "one can decide what one thinks is right, even if it doesn't seem to be the way things are done."

As a student at the University of Chicago, Volberding learned to appreciate dialectical discussions and he came to realize that progress is made as a result of logical argumentation, a principle that would serve him in later years. At the University of Minnesota Medical School he researched how viruses bind to cells by studying tumor-causing viruses in chickens. He didn't really like medicine that much. It was just a way to do science. But that changed when, as a resident in Salt Lake City, he found himself caring for a fundamentalist minister dying of cancer. The man's wife believed he could heal himself and that if he died, it would be because he had given up his faith. "I didn't know anything," Volberding said. "And I couldn't help him. No matter what I did, he was going to die." And yet, Volberding understood he could be the person the patient could turn to when no one else could help. That experience drew him to oncology and prepared him for the coming epidemic.

Volberding took a three-year fellowship at UCSF, working with cancer patients at the General and doing research in the lab of retro-virologist Dr. Jay Levy. But while working in the lab, Volberding found himself checking his watch, eager to return to his cancer patients. Lacking much of a career focus, he took the oncology job at the General.

Establishing himself as the San Francisco doctor for the new disease, Volberding was also able to keep a perspective on his patients. In those early months, he and the other straight doctors and nurses felt different from their patients. Differing sexual orientation made it easier to build defenses, not to overidentify.

The first patients they saw tended to be in their early twenties, men who had had literally thousands of sexual partners. Doctors theorized that whatever it was that was killing these men was not infectious but was something that occurred in only the most sexually active gay men. Physicians suspected that the abundance of sex and drugs, especially the sex-enhancing "poppers" (poppers is the slang term for amyl or butyl nitrite, which when inhaled, are said to intensify sexual climax), might be suppressing the patients' immune systems. Around the hospital there were lots of jokes about the patients' sexual prowess.

When he treated his patients, Volberding listened to them. If he was going to understand the disease and its causes, he knew he had to understand the gay life-style.

One of his patients, a former "queen of the Castro," the city's gay neighborhood, especially affected the oncologist. By the time the patient reached the hospital, the disease had obliterated his looks and robbed him of his body fat. On his birthday, friends brought the patient a huge birthday card that unfolded into a six-foot penis. To Volberding, the card was funny and not so funny. With a shudder, Volberding and colleagues sensed that what was going on with this man had to be related to his old life-style. And it made the doctors feel they had a responsibility to learn more.

When the man was dying, Volberding made a house call (a practice that some nurses and physicians in the outpatient AIDS clinic have continued). As the patient gasped for breath, he had around him his mother and a cluster of volunteers from an organization called the Shanti Project, which provided emotional and physical help for the dying gay men. For Volberding, the touching moment was a glimmer of what he and the others at the General could accomplish. His closeness to the former party animal leveled the wall that had divided them. The differences between gays and straights no longer meant anything. The patient was young, just like the doctor, and the patient was dying.

A black man with Pneumocystis carinii pneumonia became one of Volberding's first patients to try alternative therapies. No hospital in the country had begun drug trials. With his lover, the patient went to Israel to try an immune-system stimulator. Volberding grew close to the patient and his partner. The lover opened a newsstand in the Noe Valley neighborhood, where Dr. Volberding and his family lived. The Volberding children came to know the lover. "Then," Volberding said, "we got a chance to watch him get sick and die." Seeing people with the disease was bad enough, but seeing people he already knew developing AIDS was even worse. "If you know people before they are so sick," he said, "they're really people much more than patients."

Just when the practice of medicine was fragmenting and growing shallow, when physicians were paying more attention to profit than patients, the gay disease came along. The idealistic Volberding and the other doctors in the new field became more aware of what life was like for the patients. They came to like them and to feel a part of their deaths. "How could we not be responsive?" Volberding wondered. "How could we not try to make life as good for them as we could?" In his response, Volberding and colleagues built what has come to be called the "San Francisco Model," the finest example of humanized care for patients of the epidemic.

Initially, physicians weren't concerned about the costs of the disease. One of Volberding's early Kaposi's sarcoma patients at UCSF where he also saw patients, was a sweet, very private man suffering from intractable diarrhea and wasting. He remained in the hospital for three months. Only after his death did the doctors learn that the patient had been a member of Kaiser, a health-maintenance organization that provided its own doctors and hospitals. UCSF tried to recover the costs from Kaiser, but the HMO refused. The university ended up paying a quarter-million-dollar bill, an example, Volberding realized, of how financially devastating the disease could be. If fear hadn't dissuaded other hospitals from welcoming patients, costs would. "Institutions perked right up," Volberding said, "when they saw the potential for losses from this disease."

Yet no one could grasp the true cost or scope of it. Nor could anyone know how difficult it would be to treat. Searching for a cure, Volberding and colleagues enthusiastically investigated new treatments. Experimentation offered hope not just to dying patients but to helpless physicians as well. And as academics, the doctors were led to learn more about how to deal with the disease.

In August of 1982, Volberding and everyone else believed that alpha interferon, the first drug they tested, was going to be "The Cure." A new drug with all the aura surrounding biotechnology, alpha interferon, at least on paper, was antiviral and immuno-stimulating. With nurse Gayling Gee and a part-time high-school volunteer, Volberding recruited patients, designed consent forms and examined patients.

To design the drug test for alpha interferon, a meeting was held for the primary investigators—Volberding and Groopman and a half dozen drug-company officials in suits. All of them jammed into Volberding's tiny, out-of-the-way office—designed for a maximum of two thin people—around the desk he'd purchased at a secondhand store. When the alpha interferon group decided to take a business lunch, they relied on Volberding to recommend something suitable. They walked over to Roosevelt Tamale Parlor.

With options limited to receiving chemotherapy that had little effect, doing nothing or trying alpha interferon, the patients were eager to try the drug. Volberding had no trouble finding ten volunteers. Those ten patients made up half his caseload.

One of those patients was Dan Turner, a writer who had worked briefly as a secretary to Tennessee Williams, and who kept meticulous records in a prayer-book-size journal he wrote in each day. Turner handed over records of his sexual encounters (he had recorded the name of everyone he had ever had sex with and what they'd done together) to San Francisco's epidemiologist, Dr. Selma Dritz. Turner became one of the most famous AIDS patients in the nation, serving, in the early years, as Exhibit A, accompanying Volberding when he appeared on TV talk shows or gave speeches. With his good looks still intact, Turner considered himself the KS poster boy. (Nurse Bobbi Campbell, an early KS patient, also called himself the KS poster boy. But as Turner explained, "I was always better looking.")

Turner and the other nine human guinea pigs were so pleased to be testing alpha interferon that they gave Volberding a T-shirt with a copy of the experimental drug label on it.

The ten were treated at the hospital's Clinical Research Center inpatient research unit, a building full of patients involved in studies examining calcium balance and other dietary questions.

Early patients were seen on Thursday mornings at the University of California San Francisco. Volberding and Conant, the dermatologist (many early AIDS doctors were dermatologists who were the first to see patients with Kaposi's sarcoma), created a KS clinic, the nation's first devoted to patients with the gay cancer. But a lot of UC physicians were nervous about having gay patients with the unknown disease traipsing through the hospital, possibly exposing other patients when no one yet knew how the sickness was transmitted. Was it really safe? And did UC want to become a center for the disease?

San Francisco General was far more receptive to treating the gay men with the new disease, which by the middle of 1982 was given the name acquired immune deficiency syndrome, or AIDS. Dr. Merle Sande, chief of the medical service at the General (and vice chairman of the department of medicine at UC Medical School) gave Volberding freedom to make an offer.

Late that year, Volberding suggested moving the clinic to the General, a radical, some thought absurd, concept. The sprawling old General, a hodgepodge of dated, dark brick buildings and a newer, gray concrete one, sat in the Potrero district, an inelegant San Francisco neighborhood where gas stations nestled next to pink and yellow Victorians. The hospital stretched for several blocks, overwhelming the neighborhood. To Pulitzer Prize–winning architecture critic Allan Temko, the new gray main building resembled an ocean liner moored in a quaint old port. Altogether, the General, which also serves as a teaching hospital for UCSF, had more than five hundred beds, numerous clinics and research facilities.

The patients with AIDS, middle and upper-middle class, were not accustomed to seeking medical help from the county. Dr. Donald Abrams, one of the early AIDS doctors at UCSF, objected: "My patients all have insurance," he advised. "My patients are all intelligent, high socioeconomic-standard people. I don't want to bring them over to sit next to inmates and people that are coming in off the street." Sitting at his desk at the General, nearly a decade later, the nattily dressed Abrams says that back then he was an elitist.

Many times Volberding and Nurse Gee asked for help from Wofsy, a young infectious disease doctor, until she made it a practice to attend what she called his little clinic. As associate director of the hospital's emergency room, Wofsy was anxious to do more internal medicine. She had wearied of hospital politics and was looking for something quieter. It didn't occur to her then that her new field would grow far more political than the ER had ever been.

Later Abrams relented, bringing his patients and himself to join Volberding and Wofsy at the General. A few months passed and the university brass had changed their mind and thought that it might be a good idea to open an AIDS clinic there after all. Abrams was invited to return to head the clinic. "No," Abrams responded, "I'm no yo-yo."

Abrams, Wofsy and Volberding became medical pioneers. "No one knew anything," Volberding recalled. "But we knew more than most people." He and the other doctors were spending more and more time in medical libraries searching for articles on the opportunistic diseases with which they had no familiarity. They sought out the few other doctors in the country working on the virus, such as Groopman, then in Los Angeles. All of them were in the early stages of their careers. With no established hierarchy with which to compete, they were tossed to the forefront of the new field. And because they had become interested right way, they instantly became the closest thing to experts.

At the General, new doctors, with little sense of administration or bureaucracy, were running AIDS programs. Sometimes, programs in other cities suffered from the lack of structure and authority. But at the General the newness of the disease and the inexperience of the hospital doctors led to innovation and flexibility that came to characterize their care. That occurred, Volberding said, "mostly because we didn't know what we were doing. We didn't know what we weren't supposed to do. We didn't follow the usual rules because we hadn't been there so long that they were part of the way we operated. And that served San Francisco very well."

The doctors seemed not to know how unusual it was to have a multidisciplinary clinic that combined oncology and infectious disease and that increasingly brought in specialists. Doctors came to patients rather than the other way around. Nurses were elevated to the status of specialists, carrying their own caseloads.

Sometimes, even Volberding wondered if they were "pushing that envelope too far." Sometimes he'd try to tighten policy, but it didn't do much good. Occasionally he'd advise his graceful, gray haired, male receptionist, "We're having an important visitor tomorrow. You'll have to wear shorter earrings."

Just over a year had passed since Volberding had been visited by the twenty-two-year-old patient dying for no apparent reason. The physician anticipated having some thirty patients the following year.

In the beginning, Volberding, Abrams and Wofsy knew "every person. Then," Wofsy added, "I knew every name. Then I knew almost everybody. Then it became clear there was a second generation of AIDS patients and a third generation and a fourth and fifth. By the end of nine months, there was a group of old-timers and new recruits. By the end of nine months, we'd have a whole turnover. After the fourth generation, you couldn't begin to know the names. Then there were just a few old-timers, like Dan Turner."

If You Didn't Die, This Was Going to Be a Very Big Deal

He made his work seem almost ordinary. He was a doctor. His patients were dying. He couldn't save them. But each day he want to the hospital and did what he could. Eventually Volberding came to be seen as one of the top AIDS doctors in the world. In part his success stemmed from his behind-the-scenes maneuvers, his push for more space, his campaign for control over AIDS care in San Francisco, his charismatic presence with reporters. Beneath the easy manner and broad smiles was a diplomatic doctor-politician, a serious and ultimately victorious player. Much of his success stemmed from his decency and his own good judgment. Volberding was regularly faced with ethical, medical and political choices. Sometimes the civil rights of gay patients, or what they believed to be their civil rights, was pitted against the spread of the epidemic. Volberding and colleagues did what they thought was right. They kept doing it, even when they feared they had contracted AIDS from their patients. No test yet existed to prove them wrong.

In the beginning, no one had known enough to be afraid. As an oncologist, Volberding assumed, as others had, that the disease acted much like a regular cancer. Having just finished his oncology training, Volberding saw what he expected to see. "If you expect to see cancer and the patient has Kaposi's sarcoma, you're not going to look beyond the cancer," Volberding said. But the cancer couldn't explain how sick and wasted the patients were. KS was almost trivial, compared to the problems of the underlying disease.

There had been reports of hemophiliacs and IV drug users contracting AIDS, but nobody had yet put that together with what was happening to gay men and concluded the disease was infectious.

That changed in the autumn of 1982 when Dr. Art Ammann, the highly respected pediatric immunologist from the University of California at San Francisco Medical School, demonstrated that AIDS could be transmitted through blood. His findings were based on the case of a twenty-month-old baby, who had been born in 1981 with an Rh factor problem, requiring that his blood be exchanged. The baby had received components from nineteen blood donors from San Francisco's Irwin Memorial Blood Bank. After suffering multiple infections, the baby died in November 1982 of disseminated avium tuberculosis, a disease the body normally is able to resist. Ammann believed that the baby had not suffered from congenital immune deficiency, like the other babies he had studied, but from AIDS contracted from a blood transfusion.

He telephoned Dr. Herbert Perkins, head of Irwin Memorial Blood Bank, who put him in touch with the city's epidemiologist, Dr. Dritz. Ammann, Perkins and Dritz then examined the names of the nineteen individuals who'd supplied the blood. Dritz, who'd been keeping charts of people with AIDS and their sexual contacts, recognized the name of one donor. He'd appeared to be well when he donated the blood but by the time Dritz was examining her lists, he had already died of AIDS. The finding marked the first case anywhere in the country of AIDS being passed along in blood. It meant that the blood supplies in San Francisco, New York, Los Angeles and other cities with AIDS populations might already be AIDS contaminated.

The physicians and nurses treating AIDS patients were perfectly able to see the implications of Ammann's findings. And a shudder went through the AIDS medical community because, Volberding said, "It didn't take a genius to say, well, here I am, taking care of these patients. I now have to confront that what they have is an infectious disease." Yet they had no idea what kind of infection it was. They knew nearly nothing about its transmission. They didn't know the incubation period. They couldn't even diagnose it. Everyone was afraid he'd already gotten it.

"We knew we were still feeling well," Volberding recalled. But then, "We knew our patients had felt well before they got AIDS, too."

Sometimes at night, he awakened soaked from nightsweats, a common symptom of AIDS. In a recurring nightmare, Volberding was thinning and dying from the disease. When awake, he'd examine his skin for purplish KS lesions. When he found a blotch, colleagues had to reassure him it wasn't Kaposi's sarcoma.

Volberding was afraid all day, and sometimes he needed to come home and decompress, to say "I'm afraid," but his wife, internist Molly Cooke, was also at the hospital. She knew all too well what her husband was afraid of. And if he said, "Gee, I've got a fever. I'm afraid I have AIDS," he knew how anxiety-provoking that could be. If he was infected, Molly and their children might be, too. Or he and Molly might leave their children orphans. Cooke couldn't bear to hear him talk about it, so he had little opportunity to explain how he was feeling.

Initially Cooke had found the illness to be "a really interesting and curious disease that's obviously a disaster for the people who get it." But when they recognized the dangers involved, Cooke switched on like a light bulb. Suddenly she found it "a terrifying disease that has the potential for being a disaster for us." It made her very uncomfortable. And it gave her nightmares, too.

Everyone working in the field was frightened. Volberding was receiving calls from many of his friends such as Dr. Groopman at UCLA (now at New England Deaconess Medical Center and Harvard Medical School), who had a cough and was afraid he'd gotten AIDS. Many nurses and doctors were sure they had lymphadenopathy (enlarged lymph nodes), an early warning sign of the infection. Four times, Dr. Andrew Moss, the AIDS epidemiologist working at the General, went to his doctor to confess, "This is it, Fred. This is finally it. I'm dying."

Many others—physicians and nurses—clearly avoided working with AIDS patients. In the emergency room, gay patients or anyone thought to be gay was cocooned in paper hat, paper mask and paper gown. Food-service workers left meal trays in hallways, rather than carry them into the rooms of patients with the deadly disease. And while Cooke thought she might have been overreacting, students, interns and residents started coming to her (a role model for many, she had been the chief resident in medicine) and saying they were terrified of these patients. "People who were psychologically robust, straightforward, committed people came and said, 'I am so scared of these patients I think it's getting in the way of my taking care of them. Every night I dream I get AIDS.'"

Quitting, for Volberding, was impossible to imagine. His work was too involving, too important. Enmeshed in pioneer medicine and medical politics, he watched the disease evolve at its bedside; he cared for patients who had no place else to go, and with them he tested experimental drugs.

Volberding's colleague, Dr. John Luce, had the choice of becoming an AIDS doctor or of going into intensive-care work. He knew something was happening and he suspected "it was something you could make a career of." But Luce was more interested in treating a broader range of patients and he didn't want to get the disease. "Paul," on the other hand, "was willing to get the disease," Luce said. "He was willing to take the risk to leave the sheltered world of oncology, which is a pretty well-defined existence." That, said Luce, shows not only "a sense of adventure," but "courage." Courage, he said, "is not too strong a word."

A phlebotomist and one nurse practioner bowed out of AIDS care at the General. Full of anxiety, the rest remained. "You're going along and half of you is saying, 'You're going to die,'" said the ascerbic Moss. "The other half of you is saying, 'Well, if you're going to die, you're going to die. You may as well stay here.' If you didn't die, it was going to be a very big deal. You would become a famous scientist, as long as you were reasonably intelligent."

In America, Moss said in his clipped British accent, "people's motives have largely to do with personal ambition." So in the early years, "at least one-third of everybody's brain was saying to itself at all times, 'I'm going to be a star! If I live, I'm going to be a star.' And another third of their brains was saying, 'My God! Get me out of here! Help!' And another third of their brain was saying, 'There's a lot of sick people. We better do something.'" All three motives, he said, were operating all the time. Some doctors and nurses were higher on ambition. Others were higher on altruism.

Ever since San Francisco General had begun seeing AIDS patients, the gay men had been coming to the fifth floor of the hospital's seven-story main building, a clunky, nondescript concrete structure built in the mid-seventies that might have been a college dorm or a minimum security prison. There Volberding and Nurse Gee managed his little oncology clinic. Lacking exam tables, Volberding examined patients in beds that at night were slept in by hospital interns. (Some mornings, Nurse Gee had to awaken exhausted physicians with "Excuse me, are you ready to leave now? We're going to start clinic soon.")

Late in 1982, a pregnant medical resident asked if it was a good idea for her to sleep in the same bed that patients with the deadly disease were using during the day. No one knew the answer. But the hospital administration agreed that it might be wise to give the clinic its own space—away from everyone else.

Volberding and his expanding clinic left the central hospital, what critic Temko called "a brutal building," moving to one of what he termed the "more finely boned" old structures built when hospitals isolated patients by disease. The run-down, dark-red brick building with Spanish tiled roof, trimmed with copper gargoyles and graced with long narrow windows, stood a block and a half away from the main facility. It had all but been abandoned when the new hospital was built, but it still housed the alcohol detoxification program. Alcoholics were slouched in its hallways and stairwells. Although grateful for the space, Volberding found the interior disheartening. Rooms had been trashed. Walls were painted magenta and electric lime. The elevators were splattered with graffiti.

Armed with cans of spray paint Volberding attacked the elevator walls one weekend. A better doctor than interior decorator, the spray in the tiny space bounced off the walls onto the physician, especially when he pressed the elevator button to close the doors and tried to paint them. Sometime later he returned with Dr. Abrams and a pair of paint brushes. They repainted the elevators with a pleasant blue enamel.

Nurse Gee rummaged through the hospital's catacombs—which had been used to shoot chase scenes for the movie *Bullitt*—selecting furniture for the expanding clinic. Having found four old exam tables, some waiting-room chairs and an old metal-framed green couch, she "poured alcohol on everything and scrubbed." And with the help of a part-time high-school student to check in patients, the clinic was opened.

When they came to clean the new unit, hospital janitors wore make-shift space suits. Others observed from a distance. Epidemiologist Moss remembers the attitude. "A lot of people wanted to wait and see if we turned brown at the edges and shriveled up."

San Franciscans, like most Americans, were frightened. An AIDS patient was not allowed to sit on a San Francisco jury because fellow jurors were afraid to sit near him. Recognizing that part of his job was public education, Volberding frequently gave speeches and appeared on network and local TV. Before one morning talk show, cameramen refused to put microphones around the necks of two men with AIDS who had been invited to demystify the disease. To the TV audience, Volberding explained that there was no evidence that AIDS could be contracted through casual social contact, such as putting a microphone around someone's neck. The AIDS patients participated off camera, speaking to the audience by telephone.

The AIDS doctor turned into a talented public interpreter. Volberding's nonthreatening bedside manner and the fact that he was a heterosexual enabled him to explain the new plague to the frightened viewers and newspaper readers. With his easy manner, he seemed to slide naturally into the role of spokesman for the disease, which helped him win the unstated competition with his peers. The media needed someone who was rational and compassionate, and they didn't mind the fact that Volberding seemed to be the kind of doctor many people might want for themselves. Besides, he was approachable and cool enough to have a Grateful Dead poster in his office, although he admitted to reporters that he also enjoyed Brahms.

Journalists chronicled how he rested "a gentle hand" on a patient's shoulder and explained treatment options, letting patients make their own decisions. Such accounts reflected how far medicine had come in the fifty years from the time that doctors barely spoke to their patients at charity hospitals. And, by his example, Volberding soothed and enlightened a troubled public.

Over the years, the AIDS doctor received letters from people who had seen him on *Nightline, Merv Griffin, Donahue* or had read about him in *Time* magazine or the *International Herald Tribune*. On his office wall, Volberding has framed an envelope (sent from England) addressed and delivered to "Dr. Paul, San Francisco General Hospital, San Francisco, USA." His secretary maintains a "crank" file of letters. Many are from people alerting him to the cure: hog lard and vitamin E, milk and

Desitin ointment (from a Chicago milkman), the sap of the West African pawpaw fruit, grape juice, a half pint of sixty-proof Vodka and half a pint of Cutty Sark before bed. Other letter writers were certain that they had unraveled the cause of the disease: communism (from a San Quentin prisoner) and King Tut's tomb, where the disease had remained for two thousand years, until the King Tut exhibit came to the United States in the late 1970s. Generally, the nut letters were prefaced by such phrases as "Don't get me wrong. I'm not a nut . . ." or "I have most of my marbles . . . ." One, from London, hypothesized that AIDS was triggered by formaldehyde and "artificially generated gravity waves." Some letters were desperate cries for help. A twenty-three-page letter, describing the entire medical and sexual history of a young woman, asked if it was possible to contract the disease from a kiss. Another, from New York, asked, "Can a man take megavitamins and therefore become amune [sic] to getting herpes and or AIDS? Do Rush Me A Reply."

Despite public fears and medical warnings, the federal government was not gushing forth with AIDS research funds. In 1982, the National Cancer Institute put out a request for a proposal on AIDS. But the federal government wasn't going to speed up the normal nine-month procedure. It was, Moss felt, like some slow-moving brontosaurus: "So we're out here in San Francisco. We're wacking away at the tail. Quite a few months later, the head starts to slowly come around and pay attention." Meanwhile, Volberding, Moss and others were "going around saying "The sky is falling! The sky is falling! A lot of people are going to die.'" The federal government, they reasoned, had better do something. It didn't budge.

Following the advice of San Francisco's two most powerful gay groups, the Alice B. Toklas Memorial Democratic Club and the Harvey Milk Gay Democratic Club, Moss sought out the San Francisco board of supervisors. "Comb your hair," gay leaders advised, "and we'll get you a majority."

For three months in the spring of 1983, the epidemiologist lobbied the gay aides to the city supervisors, convincing them of the dire need for funds. Moss fit comfortably into the role of lobbyist. Before he was an epidemiologist, he'd been an antiwar activist, an editor at Ramparts Press and a writer for *Rolling Stone*. He viewed AIDS as the most political of diseases. His lobbying paid off. The supervisors came through with sixty thousand dollars for Volberding's AIDS clinic, for the Shanti

Project, which offered emotional help to lonely, dying young men, and for Moss's gay men's study, the first epidemiologic research outside the federal Centers for Disease Control. Before the vote, San Francisco Supervisor John Molinari, a sometimes mayoral candidate, declared, "I don't know what epidemiology is, but I'm going to vote for this."

"The city," Moss said, "was lovely."

While authorities at the University of California at San Francisco Medical School felt the ragtag bunch of doctors should patiently trudge through normal channels, anyone working with the disease knew of the need for money to care for patients and to begin research. If they followed protocol, more men would die without any possibility of being saved or finding out what was killing them.

In a highly unorthodox move, Dr. Conant, the dermatologist and UC's leading AIDS doctor, ignored academic and medical hierarchy, directly approaching California's assembly speaker Willie Brown, the smart, fast, powerful San Francisco state legislator. A longtime friend to the gay community, Brown told the physicians to meet in his Los Angeles office and make out their economic wish list. Some doctors sat in chairs while others spread out on the floor of Brown's office, compiling their lists. Periodically Brown would wander through the room, looking to Moss like a crafty Mephistopheles.

The legislator "liberated" (Moss's word) $2.9 million from the state budget for the University of California researchers and doctors. UC administrators appointed a task force to dole out the AIDS fund that was headed by Dr. Merle Sande, chief of medicine at the General. Appointing Dr. Sande was a little like assigning the fox to guard the henhouse. Although he was supposed to divide up the sum among the UC campuses, Sande subverted the process, funneling a large portion of it to researchers and doctors at UC Med Center in San Francisco and at San Francisco General.

Eventually the National Cancer Institute came up with the paltry sum of thirty thousand dollars. Such a pathetic amount might have discouraged some researchers. But Moss and others refused "to let the system dictate [our] priorities. This business selects people who say, 'Fuck you. Just because you won't give me any money, I'm going to do this.' People just will not allow the bureaucracy to say what their research priorities are going to be. If you're going to be a good scientist, you can't let the bureaucracy decide what the question is or how to address it. You have to ignore its attempts to sabotage you, which it will do, all the time."

The AIDS physicians fought the epidemic on numerous fronts. The general public was scared if an AIDS patient was nearby, and nonchalant if none was around, confident the disease was confined to homosexuals. But with Ammann's finding, the doctors knew better. They worried about the blood supply. Uninfected people were going to receive tainted blood.

Volberding and everyone else involved thought that only a fraction of the gay community was infected. Still, they wanted the blood banks to do something to stop the transmission of the disease through the blood supply.

Dr. Perkins, head of Irwin Memorial Blood Bank, was also worried, but the Ammann baby case was the only case in the nation that indicated that AIDS could be transmitted from a blood transfusion. Other examples existed, but none had been documented.

Perkins also worried that eliminating gay donors could drastically shrink San Francisco's blood supply (Irwin sent blood to fifty-two hospitals) and that patients would die if not enough blood was available. San Francisco's gays had long been reliable contributors to Irwin Memorial Blood Bank. A softspoken, courtly man, Perkins tried to inform the public without alarming it.

In January 1983, when fewer than two thousand people had been diagnosed with AIDS nationwide, Volberding, his mentor, Conant, and members of their Kaposi's Sarcoma Study Group wrote Irwin Memorial Blood Bank asking them to "to investigate the feasibility" of using the hepatitis B antibody test on all donated blood. Studies had shown that some 90 percent of AIDS patients also had antibodies for hepatitis.

The blood bank agreed to try the test for a month, even though Perkins said that using the hepatitis test "is not based on any rational evidence that it would screen out everyone with AIDS or anyone at all who is incubating AIDS." After trying the test for a month, Irwin Memorial quit using it.

Instead, the blood bank responded to the potential threat with a questionnaire given to all donors asking them if they had had hepatitis, AIDS, AIDS-related symptoms or if they had had multiple sex partners.

Years later, Irwin Memorial concluded that in the early eighties, one in one hundred units of its blood had been infection.

Because he had known and respected Perkins, Volberding, who is not a man to seek confrontation, said he failed to follow up the letter.

In 1984, when national medical opinion favored using the hepatitis test on blood donations, Irwin began using it again. Perkins told reporters, "We've gotten rid of a lot of eligible donors by getting rid of the gays, and we're throwing out a lot of good blood." He and others felt at the time that the risk of contracting the disease through a transfusion was "so very small," that anyone who had been transfused before the test was used "shouldn't be losing sleep over it. The biggest risk," he said, "is that people who need a blood transfusion might die because they refuse to accept it."

As patients grew frightened of the blood supply, Irwin announced that family members or other donors could not designate who would get the blood they gave. To permit such a practice would create chaos while studies had shown that the safety difference between designated blood and the general blood supply was statistically insignificant.

In September of 1984, Perkins said he was doing everything possible to see that San Francisco had the safest blood in the country.

With advances in testing, both the fear of a contaminated blood supply and the fear of contracting the disease on the job subsided. An AIDS antibody test became available that fall for research purposes. AIDS health-care workers, researchers and clerical staff at the General were tested through the labs of Dr. Jay Levy. Epidemiologist Moss did the testing, drawing his own blood last. A lot of people who took the test were positive; all were gay men. After that, fear at the General lessened.

When in March 1985 the federal government approved a commercial blood-screening test for AIDS, Irwin Memorial became the first blood bank in the nation to use it. A coalition of San Francisco's gay groups opposed its use, arguing that such a test would lead to discrimination in health insurance, jobs and housing. A press conference was held in front of a Holocaust memorial in San Francisco's Lincoln Park to dramatize the issue. Gay leaders urged blood donors to refuse the test. A humbled Perkins was not swayed by the angry gay voices.

(By 1987, Volberding and Conant stood on opposite sides of the blood controversy. Volberding defended the cautious policies instituted by Irwin. Conant argued that Irwin was wrong to wait for federal guidelines and statistics before taking action. "They have been too busy trying to reassure people that there is no problem," he declared. "If we had just said, 'We now know that there is AIDS in the blood,' lots of people might have decided against elective surgery," Conant said. "We were not informing them.")

By the early 1990s, Perkins had become aware of more than three hundred people who had contracted the AIDS virus from Irwin-supplied blood. The real numbers, he admitted, were higher. "We were in the wrong place and the wrong time," he said. "It's been an absolute horror."

But back in the mid-'80s, the doctors at the General had more than the blood supply to worry about.

You're Crazy to Come in Here

The physicians at the General knew that the illness was transmitted by blood and by sex. More and more patients continued to stream through the hospital's heavy doors. When Dr. Abrams asked them where they met their sex partners, invariably they answered, "The bathhouses."

Euphemistically named, the dozen or so San Francisco bathhouses offered an opportunity for anonymous, unprotected anal sex and other unconventional modes of intercourse with numerous partners in lavish settings such as mock Greek baths. Bathhouses operated with a city permit issued by the police department. To shut them down, the city's health director would have to declare a medical emergency.

In other cities, gay bathhouses continued unfettered. The chief of Los Angeles county's communicable disease department declared "Bathhouses don't cause AIDS, people do." In San Diego, a mayoral task force said that if the baths were to close, gay men would have to find remote places to have sex where they could not be reached with AIDS education information. In New York, the issue rarely arose. When it finally did, the city decided the bathhouses did not need regulating.

But by the spring of 1984, while the blood-bank controversy played itself out, San Francisco's baths become an issue precisely because the General's physicians were alarmed by the city sanctioned breeding grounds for AIDS. Just as they had fought to protect the blood supply, again they engaged in medical politics to close off one of the pathways for the raging epidemic.

Anxious to alert Mayor Dianne Feinstein to the public health issues, Dr. John Luce, a pulmonary specialist at the General with an early interest in AIDS, contacted her secretary, whom he'd known from Democratic Party circles. Feinstein was receptive. The two people she'd idolized most in her life had been her late father and her late second husband. Both had been physicians. Her father had been a UCSF surgeon who practiced at the General. Without any publicity, she regularly held private meetings with Sande, Volberding, Conant, epidemiologist Moss, Luce and others who taught her what they knew about the disease.

Although she relied on gay support at election time, Feinstein recognized the bathhouse issue for what it was—a medical emergency. But it occurred at a highly politicized moment. The Democratic National Convention was scheduled to meet in San Francisco that summer. A potential vice-presidential candidate, Feinstein saw to it that the cable cars, then under renovation, would be ready by convention time; that the merry-go-round in Golden Gate Park, shut down for a year, would be refurbished; that demonstrators would be allowed to demonstrate but not to disrupt. The issue of the baths could puncture an otherwise calm city.

Early in the debate, Dr. Mervyn Silverman, San Francisco's director of health, met with Volberding, Moss and other physicians from the General. At the first meeting, Moss was the only person in favor of closing the baths. He based his views on his then unpublished study showing that the more sexual partners someone had the greater was his risk of getting the disease. In long, heated debates, the group discussed the dangers of keeping the baths open versus the backlash that might occur if they were closed. Although everyone in the room was liberal,

Moss and Volberding increasingly found themselves on the "conservative" side of the issue. People's positions evolved and by the third meeting, when a straw poll was taken, the group from the General favored closing the baths.

Opposition was fierce and passionate. Silverman understood that the baths were a symbol of gay liberation. Many gay leaders, including the city's gay supervisor, Harry Britt, bath-club owners and the publishers of the gay newspapers who relied on the baths for much of their advertising revenue, claimed closing them was a violation of their civil rights and was not based on medical evidence.

Mayor Feinstein shot back that the only civil right involved was the questionable right to commit suicide. A few gay leaders sided with her. They were labeled self-hating homophobes.

It was true that at the time no one had proven that the disease was sexually transmitted. It was only a very, very strong medical assumption. Many, such as Moss, Abrams and Volberding were willing to accept it as proven. The baths had become death houses. They had to be shut down. But gay leaders said that if the baths were boarded up, the gay bars would be next, then the gay businesses and gay clubs.

In the city's health director, gay activists found an ally. As the only official with the power to close the baths, Silverman argued that the city would be better served to leave them open. Gays had to alter their own behavior, not have it dictated to them. His position was part medical, part public health, part sociological. What was happening, he contended, was more important than where it was happening. Shut the baths, he claimed, and anonymous gay sex with multiple partners would continue elsewhere. Better to leave the baths open and educate the customers, than to crawl around park rose bushes looking for men to teach them safe sex. If gays fled the baths themselves, Silverman argued, the impact would affect the entire gay community. In his attempt to educate, he ordered the baths to post signs warning about AIDS. Signs were indeed posted—in darkened hallways.

In their earnest, naïve way, the AIDS doctors thought that perhaps the problem could be solved by educating the bathhouse owners. Volberding and colleagues invited the entrepreneurs to the hospital. When Volberding learned that the bathhouse owners arrived with their lawyers, he suspected the meeting was not going to go as well as planned. In the hallway outside, a TV reporter trolled for a story.

The owners expressed their concern for AIDS. They tried to engage the physicians in an extensive discussion on the safety of Crisco versus other lubricants. They talked about hand-washing facilities, additional lighting and condoms. They offered to remove cushions from the orgy rooms.

Eager to avoid a them-versus-us feeling, the doctors talked about mutually gaining control over the disease.

Volberding had brought along his carousel of AIDS slides to teach the businessmen AIDS 101. The bathhouse owners weren't buying. They hadn't come to look at dying customers. "Don't give us that stuff," one said. Their livelihood was being challenged by these overeager doctors. One of the owners barked: "Let's be realistic. We're both in this for the money. We're here to make money from their sex and you're here to make money from their disease."

Volberding ended the meeting abruptly.

Over the following months, the controversy intensified as it became more obvious that the baths would not close voluntarily and that gay men were continuing to frequent them despite warnings that such visits could kill them.

Health director Silverman felt pulled by all sides. The mayor, he said, "wanted me to do what there was no political will to do." He considered her approach "simplistic." "Sex and Dianne," he said, "are two very distant things . . . . "She spent most of her time talking about the wonders of celibacy. She was," he joked, "orgiastic about it."

One of San Francisco's most astute older politicos advised Silverman to "maker her happy, just close them." Silverman would not give in.

But Moss, Wofsy, Volberding and Abrams were seeing the parade of bathhouse graduates at the General. "I am not a guilt-driven person," Volberding said some years after the controversy, "but I have felt that I personally should have done more in the bathhouse issue. We were doing a lot: meetings after meetings. There certainly was a time when we knew damn well this virus was being transmitted in the bathhouses. Jesus, it didn't take a genius to know that. The idea that people were going to places of business; they were advertising themselves; people were being encouraged to go . . . . We should have been out there with banners ourselves at night saying YOU'RE CRAZY TO COME IN HERE!"

AIDS policy was being formulated weekly at the Thursday meetings of UCSF physicians (also General doctors), health director Silverman and city epidemiologist Selma Dritz. Chaired by Sande and Volberding, the group was forced to make policy before its members knew much about the disease. They discussed private rooms for AIDS patients, protective eyewear for health-care workers and cardiopulmonary resuscitation. But when they broached the bathhouse issue, their collegial consensus disintegrated.

After months of meetings, health director Silverman told Feinstein and the doctors he would shut the bathhouses down.

The night before the press conference at which the announcement was to be made, Silverman went to a gay cabaret to confer with more than one hundred people from the local gay papers and the baths. He had been told that the gay leadership had signed a petition supporting the closure. Their sudden conversion was caused by one gay activist who was threatening to put the bathhouse issue on the November ballot. Gay leaders believed the public would vote to shut them. But before Silverman reached the meeting, the names of the leaders had been leaked to the gay press and they were accused of being traitors. By the time the meeting began, most of the leaders had removed their signatures.

The next day, Silverman was an hour late for his own press conference. When he appeared, he was wearing a bulletproof vest and was accompanied by three plainclothes policemen. His life had been threatened the day before. He apologized but said he was not ready to make a decision. While local and national media watched, he refused to take any questions.

In October 1984, saying that the disease "evidently is a sexually transmitted viral disease," the health director finally ordered the closing of the baths. "Like putting a sign up that 'Sugar is bad for you,' in a candy store," Silverman said, "we found out [educating customers at the baths] wasn't working."

The bathhouse owners took the city to court. A judge ordered the baths reopened with monitors ordered to check on patrons at ten-minute intervals.

In time, patronage dwindled. The controversy, which was covered in newspapers and television newscasts, had led to a massive educational campaign. The bathhouses closed for lack of business. "As more and more gay men lost friends and lovers to AIDS," said city epidemiologist Dritz, "the lesson was learned in the most tragic way."

Although he was no public health expert, Volberding said, he felt strongly that "something was responsible for this epidemic and that we had our own responsibility to speak out."

In the General's hospital beds, men in their twenties kept dying. The American public still clung to the cheery hope that a cure would be found soon. Doctors and researchers knew better. Frantically they searched for something, even unconventional solutions, to slow the development of the disease.

The Results Had to Be Wrong

During the fall of 1986, a Hong Kong doctor traversed the United States with a briefcase full of herbal remedies. He'd gone to the National Institutes of Health, but no one would see him. He'd stopped at the University of California at Davis, where he'd hit it off with Dr. Robert Chang, who promised to test his concoctions for anti-HIV (Human Immunodeficiency Virus) activity. The Davis professor's findings were later published in an obscure plant-science journal that no one in the AIDS community seemed to have read.

Now, in old red-brick Building 80 at San Francisco General, where most of the AIDS activity was centered, the small doctor walked past the multicolored poster board listing medical services in nine languages. He boarded the temperamental elevator so full of recent immigrants (on their way to the refugee health clinic) and AIDS patients that it often

34

recalled Rockwell's painting of peoples of the world. This was the nearly abandoned building Volberding had expropriated for his AIDS clinic. By autumn 1986, it was foaming with activity. Unheralded, the man from Hong Kong arrived on Ward 84. Dr. Hin-Wing Yeung was looking for a receptive physician and a number of human guinea pigs with AIDS. Yeung brought his ancient herbal remedies and new-age business acumen, with an accent on the acumen. Scanning the black-and-white wall directory, he found what he was searching for: a Chinese surname. He went to the front desk and asked to see Dr. Gifford Leoung, then a thirty-three-year-old AIDS doctor.

The Hong Kong scientist possessed grandiose plans, but he was stymied in his lab. With only three known HIV-positive patients then in Hong Kong he might as well have been peddling windshield wipers in the Sahara; he had no one on whom to test his theory. A protein biochemist, Yeung was director of the Chinese Medicinal Material Research Center at the Chinese University of Hong Kong. If he was going to do in vivo testing, it would have to be done elsewhere.

"I have something I think will inhibit the growth of HIV," Yeung told the young San Francisco AIDS doctor.

"I'm not sure why you want to speak with me," Leoung replied.

"I want you to give it to patients and see how it works," Yeung explained matter-of-factly. He hadn't yet heard about the Food and Drug Administration, animal toxicology studies and drug protocols. He didn't understand drug testing's glacial melt. Instead, he saw it simply. People were dying. He had a drug that might cure them. Why not try it on them?

What was to become known as Compound Q might never have made it to America had it not been for Dr. Leoung's respect for Chinese medicine. He did not dismiss the Hong Kong scientist as a kook in a suit bearing garlic, tree bark or other folk remedies.

Leoung, who would become the principal investigator of aerosolized pentamidine, a prophylatic treatment developed at San Francisco General Hospital that has kept thousands of AIDS patients free from PCP (Pneumocystis carinii pneumonia), the deadly AIDS pneumonia, was receptive. He viewed AIDS research like the American space program; a lot of what scientists would discover would help people in genetics, chemistry, cellular biology and in other fields of medicine. Although he worked with patients and not test tubes, Leoung looked for ways to help the scientist from Hong Kong. After explaining to Yeung about the FDA and drug testing, he said, "I know someone who might be able to help you."

The two men walked down the busy corridor to the reception desk. Just then, the elevator door parted. Out strode the gregarious Dr. Michael McGrath.

A strapping Irishman, McGrath is an immunobiologist with an MD and a Ph.D. At thirty-four, he was head of the AIDS Immunobiology Research Lab at the hospital. The popular German magazine *Bunte* would later describe him as looking more like a "baseballstar" (*sic*) than a man juggling petri dishes. Tall, with a wide, friendly face and brown curly hair with flecks of gray he earned in medical school, McGrath was Tom Sawyer in a lab coat. When he peered into a microscope others wanted to see what he saw.

To the growing East Coast AIDS establishment, he was a California whippersnapper. A UC researcher for only one year, he'd plunged into his work, testing various remedies.

McGrath paused, but only momentarily. His propensity for talking to anyone who engages him goes against the more circumspect diplomacy of modern science. At times it put him in an awkward position with his colleagues. Yet rarely did he turn anyone down.

"Okay," he said, bridging continents; he was willing to talk to Yeung.

The smaller man accompanied McGrath down the elevator, across the street and to his lab, a crowded island on the third floor of a building almost nobody could find without a compass.

Yeung told about his concoction that he said could inhibit the growth of HIV. The classic Chinese approach to disease is to treat illness with multiple mixtures of extracts cooked into a tea and taken for a short period of time. The belief is that the interplay of the extracts benefits the patient. McGrath listened, but multiple extracts did not appeal to him. Too many variables. A mixture could contain thousands of components. McGrath was a scientific speed freak. He couldn't tolerate the potential research lagging on for years.

With charts, chalk and board, he gave Yeung a quick-hit class in AIDS—McGrath style. AIDS, he said, is a disease of infected macrophages. Back then, his assertion was not yet part of the accepted wisdom on AIDS. Even two years later, Dr. Anthony Fauci, director of the National Institute of Allergy and Infectious Diseases, still claimed T cells, the white blood cells most important in fighting viral infection and cancers, were the major source of the virus. People die from their loss of

T cells, McGrath agreed, but it is the smoldering infection of macrophages that he believed caused T cells to become infected and die.

Macrophages are the common immune-system cells found in the brain, lungs, liver, spleen, bone marrow and virtually every organ of the body. They gobble up infectious agents and signal T cells that a foreign invader is coming. In his in vitro work at the lab, McGrath and researchers had concluded that these scavenger cells were the reservoir of HIV infection. T cell death, they argued, was secondary. McGrath told his visitor he was looking for a toxin that could kill infected macrophages.

"Ohhhhh. I know something that kills macrophages," Yeung said.

"Great, that's fantastic," McGrath said with the enthusiasm of a kid finding glow-in-the-dark planets in his cereal box. "When you go back to Hong Kong, why don't you send me some? I'd be real happy to test it out and see if it just kills macrophages or whether there's selective killing of infected cells."

The Hong Kong scientist went away. A couple of hours later he returned, popped open his briefcase and pulled out two vials of homemade white powder: extract of trichosanthin, the root of a Chinese cucumber plant, and extract of momorcharin, from the seeds of Chinese bitter melon.

From this encounter would come two and a half years of research so secret that the *Village Voice* later described it as comparable to the Manhattan Project. Other possible panaceas had come and gone, but none would have the appeal of the milligram of white powder in Yeung's vial. The Chinese scientist was enthusiastic. The American was skeptical but open to experimentation.

That was always part of the appeal of science for McGrath. By the time he was a sophomore at the University of Minnesota the lab had become his sandbox. While studying chicken leukemia, trying to figure out how the virus infects cells, he found his life's work. (While a medical student at the university, Volberding worked on McGrath's study.) "Here's something that's so interesting to do and there are people who will pay you to do it. You can try to figure out how something works and actually make progress. That's the hook. Do it and if you don't find anything, well, that's not any fun," he says with a laugh. "It's the first, second, third unique finding. It just sinks the hook in."

He'd grown up the only son of a business administrator for a Minnesota correctional institution. His uncle, a doctor, was the family icon.

His cousins went into medicine. As an excellent student, he figured he could, too.

His excitement over AIDS research and his belief in the importance of macrophages was contagious. Although tiny, his lab at the General became a bustling quarter of young researchers. Classical music alternating with rock wafted through the room. Counter space was cluttered with beakers, papers and (with so little floor space) somebody's ten-speed.

It used to be that McGrath worked in the lab seven days a week because he loved his work and because he couldn't think of a reason not to. But after his wife, Deborah, who became the General's director of nursing for medicine, gave birth to their first child, he began spending weekends at home. Given the constraints of a well-balanced life, McGrath was still a fast-tracker. In time, AIDS activists would pressure him. And the pure scientist, so apolitical that he wasn't a registered voter, would be forced to consider the link between his petri dishes, politics and the dying young men. In time, he would be forced to choose between scientific silence and cooperating with AIDS activists. When information about the Chinese protein was made public, some HIV-positive people at the hospital groused that McGrath's findings would have come sooner if he'd been a desperate AIDS patient instead of a healthy heterosexual with a happy family.

In many ways, AIDS was the perfect disease for him. He talked fast, thought fast and liked fast answers. "I'm not a plodder. So you say, if you want the results quickly of research into human disease, what kind of disease do you work on? Do you want to work on something that takes twenty or thirty years to kill somebody? Heart disease? Kidney disease? Or do you want something that kills people quickly so that if you make a fundamental discovery or breakthrough you can apply it and you'll know the answer quickly? Because of my personality, I like to know the answer to things. You look at human disease and say, 'What kills people quickly?' Cancer does. And the type of cancer I work on, especially lymphomas. AIDS lymphomas are horrible! Mean survival of AIDS lymphomas are three to four months."

With trichosanthin he expected quick answers, too. If it worked in the body, it would work quickly. If it failed, he'd know that quickly, too. His own speed, however, wasn't as intense as that of AIDS activists, who were willing to try untested drugs rather than try nothing at all.

Many scientists spend their lab hours filling cracks in other people's research. Their labs are devoted to discovering details of larger matters that are understood. McGrath was too bold, too anxious. With his rat-tat-tat laugh, he explained, "We look for the biggest pile of dogma and step on it. You get criticized by the ninety percent of the people who established that dogma. That's been the story of my scientific career.

"I don't kiss anybody's ass," he said—not on the East Coast and not at the General. That openness and antiestablishment attitude probably made him more amenable to considering Eastern medicine.

That attitude, however, was not conducive to rising in the structured world of academia. As with Volberding, if McGrath was going to deal with AIDS, and in his case with herbal medicine, he would be going out on an academic limb. Some of his peers began questioning his objectivity. Many took a colder view of what was happening, and they thought that most of the drugs being looked at "were garbage and most of the patients [who believed in them] were fooling themselves," as one colleague put it.

Before McGrath encountered Yeung, he was engaged in more traditional research, trying to prove that macrophages were the reservoir of AIDS. His first few grant applications implicating macrophages "were murdered." The prevailing attitude and one that appeared on the pink sheets, the commentaries for grants, said, "Why work on macrophages? Everyone knows macrophages have nothing to do with AIDS."

McGrath had learned how to buck adversity years before. As a teenage gymnast, he'd grown accustomed to failure—in nine out of ten initial attempts, a gymnast falls off his apparatus. Unlike a player in team sports, a gymnast had only himself to blame for mistakes. One year he shot up six inches, making it even harder for the six-foot-two athlete to compete. He could have switched to basketball had there not been extenuating circumstances: he played too rough and he couldn't make baskets. So he stuck with gymnastics. Sitting in his lab he drew parallels with his work. "Science is hammering away at a problem and having failure after failure after failure and not giving up and gradually changing things so that you can increase your chance of success."

Adversity only fueled him. Yeung had something he claimed killed macrophages. But the research was problematic. As natural adhesives, macrophages glom onto glass and plastic like nature's own superglue. This characteristic makes it difficult for scientists to quantify experiments. And it made it impossible for McGrath and colleagues to observe what happened after macrophages become infected with HIV. Research was stymied until Dr. Suzanne Crowe, working in McGrath's lab, hit upon a solution. She had introduced lab researchers to walnut oil and balsamic vinegar for their kitchens, and now she introduced the lab to the wonders of Teflon. Like ham and eggs, macrophages don't stick to Teflon. With Teflon dishes, Crowe was able to culture macrophages and sample them over weeks and months. For the first time, she could quantify the degree of HIV in macrophages. Observing over time, Crowe showed that, unlike T cells that become infected with HIV and die, macrophages get infected and stay infected. In the test tube, at least, macrophages were continuous production factories of HIV.

By 1987, McGrath's thinking wasn't considered far out any longer. Researchers in the lab of Dr. Robert Gallo, the leading scientist at the National Cancer Institute, became backers of macrophages as the major player.

Having decided how AIDS broke down the immune system, McGrath set about to fix it. He began looking for things that might kill HIV-infected macrophages or lessen the expression of HIV in the macrophages. The fatal flaw for macrophages is that they'll eat anything. Their Latin name means "big eater." In an experiment conducted many years ago, mice were injected with very fine ground glass. Macrophages ate the glass, and every macrophage in the mice's bodies was killed. Their ability to eat anything is one of the ways that macrophages fight off viruses, infections and bacteria in the body.

Given macrophages' appetite, McGrath decided to dress up a little poison, so that it could reach macrophages without dispersing toxins elsewhere in the body. Utilizing a Trojan Horse approach, he decided to load up fat globules known as liposomes with toxins. Theoretically, at least, the poison enveloped in the fat globule would not kill anything but the targeted macrophages. Only the macrophages would eat up the globules and the toxins would do their job and kill the macrophages.

You can kill off the macrophages in mice, as the glass did, and within a few weeks, bone marrow, which produces macrophages, will have resupplied the body with more.

Unlike many of his peers, McGrath never viewed AIDS from the more accepted infectious-disease perspective of blocking the spread of the virus. AZT, the first drug approved for the treatment of AIDS, only blocked the virus but did nothing about already infected cells. He preferred "the sledgehammer approach." Kill off every infected macrophage and hope it doesn't kill the person. "That sounds sort of brutal," he admitted, "unless you follow what oncologists do for a living. They kill hundreds of billions of cells." Trained as a hematologist, McGrath had no problem declaring war on the body.

He was looking for the right toxin to envelop in the liposomes when Yeung appeared. Yeung had spent the last seven years in his lab purifying and characterizing trichosanthin and momorcharin, mostly working on the latter. In China, these plant proteins had been used for centuries to induce abortions.

Trichosanthin is from the Trichosanthes kirilowii plant that grows only in China. When the protein purified from the plant's root is injected into pregnant women, it causes placental death and abortion. In China about one hundred thousand women use it each year. Trichosanthin had also been one of the main drugs used to treat metastatic choriocarcinoma, a malignancy of the placenta. The disease spreads throughout the body—just like HIV disease.

So McGrath began experimenting with the white powders from Hong Kong. Periodically the Chinese scientist sent the American suspicious-looking glassine envelopes of white powder. At times, McGrath wondered if he'd be arrested as part of an international cocaine cartel. To conduct his experiments, McGrath couldn't use normal T cells, which die when infected with HIV. Instead, he used other cell lines that continuously replicate the virus without keeling over. He added trichosanthin to these infected cells. Four days out he could detect no virus replication.

McGrath felt it had to be wrong. "It was very interesting, very potent," he said, "but it had to be wrong." If you treated infected cells with AZT, nothing would happen. If you treated infected cells with trichosanthin the virus replication stopped. With the Chinese extract, researchers could no longer detect HIV proteins. No other drug performed so well. McGrath did another experiment and another. He and his researchers did almost a half year's worth of test-tube experiments. They thought that what they were finding was some giant artifact. Yet the results didn't deviate. In science, if something appears to be impossible, it probably is. McGrath could think of no good biochemical or biophysical reason for the extract to be so effective.

In the beginning, his assay system was set up to look at the infected cells at day five. Trichosanthin or what McGrath nicknamed Q, for the Chinese cucumber, quickly eliminated virus replication, but it took ten to fifteen days before it went on to kill infected cells. It was two years before McGrath found that infected cells treated with Q went on to die. "Why does it only kill infected cells really, fairly exclusively? I mean how could we design a drug to do that? The answer is, I haven't a clue—right now."

McGrath knew that Q's performance in a petri dish might not be replicated in the human body. As a plant protein, Q was a toxin. The human body couldn't absorb it forever. Yet its effect in vitro was stunning. Although too early to consider the possibilities, the numbers could not be ignored. If Q worked, it could save thousands of lives. If not, it was just another dud, or worse, deadly. Still, nothing tested so far had performed as well as Yeung's white powder.

For months, McGrath and his collaborators at Genelabs, the drug lab that contracted with Yeung to manufacture Q, conducted their quiet experiments. McGrath thought like a scientist, unaware of how his discovery would be perceived by the people it was designed to save.

Call Her Selfless, Decent and Caring

On May 22, 1987, the twenty-four-year-old nurse's first day at San Francisco General, the federal Centers for Disease Control issued a troubling report. Three more health-care workers had been infected with the AIDS virus while on the job.

"How long before my mother calls?" she kiddingly asked coworkers, while continuing her duties. In the days before she'd stuck herself with a needle full of AIDS blood, she had felt invulnerable.

The call came, as she knew it would. A loving, kind woman, her mother promised not to lecture. She told her daughter she supported her in her work. She just wanted to warn her. The daughter understood. From a good Catholic family, the daughter knew how her mother felt: a woman's greatest gift from God was the gift of a child. AIDS could destroy it.

The CDC's weekly *Morbidity and Mortality Report* described three incidents: one worker had had a small amount of blood on her index finger for twenty minutes; the second, a phlebotomist filling a vacuum tube with blood, was splashed with blood on her face and in her mouth; and the third, a medical technologist, had blood spilled over most of her hands and forearms. The report said that the first worker had chapped hands; the third had had dermatitis on an ear and might have scratched it. Critics would say later that the CDC underplayed the danger, not wanting to frighten health-care workers. Its report concluded: "The three cases reported here suggest that exposure of skin or mucous membranes to contaminated blood may rarely result in transmission of HIV."

The three incidents brought the reported number of American health-care workers who had contracted the AIDS virus on the job to nine. The real figures were higher, although no one knew how high. Many workers would not report a needle-stick. Some refused to be tested. Others failed CDC's stringent standards requiring that they have been tested for AIDS before they seroconverted, which meant before their blood began to show antibodies to the AIDS virus.

A few days later, San Francisco General proposed extending its body-substance precautions to all patients because no one could know for sure who was going to be HIV positive. A lot of health-care workers might balk, but gloves and other protective gear were going to have to be worn when dealing with blood or other bodily fluids from any patient.

Safer, better-engineered equipment was becoming available. Just about the time that the new nurse arrived at the hospital, a salesman was seen striding from one unit to the next, dumping samples of safer needles that could prevent many sticks. The equipment was deemed prohibitively expensive.

Although the nurse had always excelled in science and could have scrambled to become a doctor, she loathed competition. On the morning of her SATs, she awakened thinking about her future and determined then that she would rather be a nurse. It was not an informed decision. She had little idea of what she was getting into. She'd never worked in a hospital and she didn't know any nurses. But she did well in health sciences and she liked working with people. At the age of eleven, she had helped care for and feed a first-grader with muscular dystrophy. When the child died, the nurse-to-be was devastated. In high school, she had helped the toy drive and had organized activities for the elderly at a nearby nursing home.

It was part of a continuum. By the time she reached San Francisco, she had lost none of her sense of decency. When almost everyone else had hardened to downtown beggars, she'd spot one, make eye contact, unzip her bag and plunk money in a needy hand. It wasn't enough to work with AIDS patients; every week she also volunteered at a soup kitchen. Her MasterCard depicted a pastel image of a girl running in a field of flowers. It was from Sane Freeze, an organization opposed to the proliferation of nuclear weapons. But call her selfless, decent, caring, and she would slough off the compliment with self-mockery and a laugh.

Right out of nursing school she had worked at an affluent private New York hospital. One of her supervising nurses there sensed that she had a different calling. "I know you may not be very comfortable working here," the older woman observed. "Nursing is more than a job for you." The nurse felt that before that supervisor she was standing naked. In fact, the new nurse held nothing against rich patients who wanted their every need attended to, she just felt she could do much more.

She left New York for San Francisco where she waited five months for the job at the General. While a hiring freeze remained in effect, she worked at other area hospitals. Then in the spring of 1987, she landed a job at the General. Work would be hard, but it would be real.

During orientation, she was impressed with the emphasis the hospital placed on infection control. They taught her how to safely use equipment, where to place waste and how to operate syringes that required less manipulation than others. Yet the onus for safety still fell on the nurses themselves. Slow down, she was told. Prioritize. It sounded good, but it was unrealistic. When have nurses learned to prioritize themselves over a patient? the nurse wondered.

Shortly after she began work, the young nurse enlisted in the hospital's AIDS health-care workers study. "In the name of science," she was tested. Dr. Julie Gerberding's research included some one thousand persons—eight hundred of them from San Francisco General. An assistant professor of medicine at University of California Medical School in San Francisco, the no-nonsense Gerberding arrived at the hospital about the same time as the epidemic. She coped with her fears through scientific method and research, designing the largest AIDS health-care workers study in the nation.

Three tubes of the young nurse's blood were drawn. To test for HIV an ELISA test was conducted at two labs—one at the University of California at Davis and the other in top AIDS researcher Levy's lab at the UCSF. Short for Enzyme Linked ImmunoSorbant Assay, the test could detect small amounts of antibodies to the virus. Two labs were used to avoid mislabeling. As with others participating in the study, some of her blood serum was stored at the UCSF's serum and tissue bank. She felt certain it would never be needed.

She already knew her test results: Negative.

Her mother may have worried about needle-sticks and blood splashes, but the nurse was too pleased with her new job to be much concerned, even though needle-sticks are a common occupational hazard. At a conference seminar on nursing and AIDS that same year (sponsored by the hospital) members of the audience were asked to raise their hands if they had ever been stuck by a needle. Nearly everyone in the room raised a hand. AIDS had added a surrealistic atmosphere to the General. "It's the stuff of breakfast, lunch and dinner," one nurse confided. Many were intimidated by it. Some people quietly moved to country hospitals to avoid caring for HIV-positive patients. A few changed careers. One nurse who quit patient care explained his reasoning: "A carpenter bangs his thumb. An accountant makes a mistake on his spread sheet. A nurse sticks himself. The carpenter may get a bruise. The accountant might lose his job. The nurse might be killing himself."

New nurses and physicians seemed especially vulnerable. Although well trained, they had to adjust to cumbersome equipment and the rush that comes with understaffing.

By the time the new nurse had been hired, employee health was seeing four or five hospital workers each week who had stuck themselves with needles or other sharp instruments and were worried about contracting AIDS. None had. Maybe, in retrospect, the doctors and nurses were suffering from denial, from a belief that it couldn't happen here. They grew up with antibiotics, vaccines and a sense that most illnesses could be treated. Older clinicians remembered the risks of contracting polio and tuberculosis. But science had made modern medicine safe. At least that was the agreed-upon myth.

Gerberding's early data and companion studies around the country led the doctor to conclude that the risks were low. Only nine months earlier, a UPI story based on her findings stated: "Hospital workers did not catch AIDS even when they were accidentally jabbed with needles or splashed in the face with blood from patients infected with the deadly illness, researchers said." Out of twenty-four hundred health-care professionals in various studies, only one had contracted the disease. "The basic message," Gerberding told the reporter, "is that no special controls are needed."

She said that before the young nurse stuck herself.

Maybe It Was Mono

The nurse had stuck herself on an early summer's morning. She knew that other nurses had stuck themselves, even with the blood of HIV-positive patients. And nothing had happened to them. Such accidents were bound to occur. By 1987 an estimated one-fourth of all the patients showing up for care at the General were carrying the AIDS virus. Still, it was a little unsettling.

After she stuck herself, the nurse followed procedures the hospital had implemented for health-care workers with needle-sticks. She went to employee health. There they worried not so much about AIDS as about hepatitis B, another occupational hazard for health-care workers. The CDC estimates that some two hundred health-care workers die each year from acute or chronic consequences of hepatitis B they acquire on the job. But hepatitis B has never been feared the way AIDS has because the disease is preventable by vaccine, the time between exposure and (in the small percentage of cases) death is twenty to thirty years, and hepatitis B isn't stigmatizing the way AIDS is.

The nurse thought little more about the stick and returned to work. Five days later she spiked a fever that lasted two days. Then she had another fever for a week. Debilitated, she lost her appetite and suffered muscle aches. Again, the flu went away. A few days later, the fever returned. For four weeks, the nurse lay in bed, ill and, because she was so new on the job, unpaid. She crawled to the bathroom and crawled back. Having moved out from the East Coast only recently, she hardly knew anyone in San Francisco, much less a doctor.

In the middle of her illness, she found a doctor with a Marcus Welby manner. She told him about the needle-stick and the flu. Reassuringly, he told her not to worry. But her flu wasn't improving. She suspected she had mononucleosis.

The dramatic illness persisted. Frightened, one night she telephoned the doctor's office again. Instead of reaching Marcus Welby, she talked with his partner, an analytical icicle. She walked in and was about to ask for a test for mono when he said, "Perhaps you've seroconverted," which would mean she would be developing antibodies in her blood to the AIDS virus, a sign that she was HIV positive. "Wouldn't it be interesting to put you on AZT?"

He scared the hell out of the nurse.

At the hospital, clinical nurse specialist Rita Fahrner was becoming concerned, too. Although it was not widely known, AIDS specialists recognized that when someone became HIV positive, he frequently became ill with flulike symptoms weeks afterward that eventually disappeared.

Fahrner consulted Gerberding, the head of the hospital's AIDS health-care workers study. The doctor thought it unlikely that anyone would fall ill only five days after exposure. If she believed the nurse might have been infected, she would have considered putting her on the health-care workers AZT study. Sponsored by its makers, Burroughs Wellcome, the study was designed to give health-care workers AZT immediately after exposure. The hope was that the drug might halt the virus from reaching the DNA of cells, thereby preventing infection. Having seen hundreds of exposed nurses and doctors of whom not one had acquired the virus, Gerberding was optimistic. Still, she and Fahrner both felt the nurse should take the AIDS test.

Four weeks after the needle-stick, the nurse had her blood drawn. The blood was sent to Levy's lab for an immunofluorescent assay (IFA) (a highly sensitive test), a Western Blot and an antigen test.

The antigen test, which measures proteins specific to the virus, came back positive. The IFA was borderline. The Western Blot was negative. Gerberding wasn't sure what these results meant. The antigen test was new and she had had little experience with its accuracy. There was no firm evidence of HIV antibodies in the nurse's blood.

The nurse was told the testing had been inconclusive. She would have to come in six days later to give more blood for still more tests. This time, she was given the ELISA, which detects antibodies to HIV, IFA, Western Blot and antigen tests. The flu disappeared; the young nurse returned to work.

The scare had matured her. Suddenly she was thinking about life and appreciative of her good health. Once again she felt fine. The stick, the first she'd ever had, had been a warning.

She waited for her test results.

The French Kiss

On a Saturday morning in September 1987, her doorbell rang.

The young nurse threw open the window sash and looked to the sidewalk. A fragile-looking woman with a perpetually sad face stood below. The head nurse, her boss.

Was I doing a lousy job or what? the young nurse thought. If the woman had come by in the afternoon, maybe the young nurse could explain away her visit, but something about the morning was so specific.

Part of her knew. Her boss really didn't even have to come in.

The woman climbed the steps to the little apartment. An efficiency, the room was cluttered with a big bed and an ironing board that doubled as a table. An orange cat moseyed about. Pictures of family and friends were on the refrigerator door.

The younger woman arranged her pair of frayed upholstered chairs so that the two could face one another. Her boss was distraught. She had to relay the worst information she could possibly relay—and it was to her newest employee, the baby of the unit.

The needle-stick. The blood. The virus. But she thought she'd squeezed it all out right then. The tests. The healthy younger woman, her life before her, heard the words. She was HIV positive. After the second round of tests, her ELISA came back positive. The more sensitive IFA test returned positive. And the antigen and Western Blot were also positive. (The first Western Blot test, which had been interpreted as negative, had shown P 24 band, which she later learned is the first to appear when someone is seroconverting.) About six weeks after the accident her blood was showing clear evidence of seroconversion. The AIDS virus was roaming around inside her.

At first, she failed to respond. In that moment, the entire face of the world changed. Her innocence was shattered.

They talked. She kiddingly said, "Thanks, you just took fifty years off my life." She was only twenty-five. Then her boss left.

The conversation had lasted twenty minutes. If it hadn't been for the position of the chairs, she would not have believed it had happened.

The truth plunged her into a dreamlike state. She paced the small floor. She felt empty. She knew she should call someone. Who? She'd have to be more together before laying it on her parents. Her brother was taking the Graduate Record Exams. She didn't want to ruin his concentration. She couldn't call an old friend living nearby. The friend was so petrified of AIDS she refused to eat in restaurants in the gay Castro district. The nurse called Regina, her best friend, in Minnesota. The friend became hysterical, announcing she'd fly in by Monday.

That day and the next, the nurse who would come to be known throughout the hospital and the city of San Francisco as Jane Doe, walked a lot. She walked along Market Street through its gay sector and its seedy parts. Past the big women's clothing stores, the shops with cheap, lavender organdy little girls' dresses, past the McDonald's and the Jack-in-the-Box and the Taco Bell that make the wide avenue almost Anyplace, USA. When she passed Grand Central Antiques she considered how comforting some furniture might be. Then she thought "Why bother?" Sometimes she felt like she was she was swimming underwater. She'd never done hard drugs, but she imagined they might make you feel the way she felt. Everything was distorted, out of focus.

She felt awful. Yet as calamities go, she felt she'd lucked out. She still had all her limbs. As she walked along Market Street she kept reminding herself, I can dance! I can dance! I can dance!

The night before Regina arrived, Jane Doe went for a drive across the Golden Gate Bridge and to dinner in elegant Marin County with Jonathan, a nurse with whom she'd been close. Afterward, they strolled outside, and in the dark Jane Doe screamed: "I'm going to be dying! And everybody's going to be processing their feelings. There'll be all this conflict-resolution. Everyone will feel better. There'll be a memorial service with meaningful music and liturgy. Everyone will feel purged! Everyone will feel better! They'll go off and have sex! I'll still be dead, fucking dead!"

Then she turned to Jonathan and inquired, "We've been teaching safe sex. Do you really think you can't get it from French kissing? We teach it but do you really believe it?"

His answer was definitive. And in the kiss, her healing began.

"Irish Catholics should not be allowed to have HIV," she said later. "What are the two things this culture doesn't deal with? Death and sex. I don't mean to be disparaging, but we have trouble in these two areas. Now they're linked. It shouldn't be allowed!"

Spirited, smart, funny, sweet. Jane Doe's basic character could not be crushed by the bulldozer of diseases. The diagnosis only exaggerated what was. She came to believe that "HIV is a chemical reaction with who you are."

That first week, Jane Doe, Regina and Jonathan did a lot of dancing. They went to Rocking Robins, a dance club that plays oldies. She skipped work for four days and danced all night. It was not unlike an Irish Catholic wake, where people drift off to the haystacks and make love. She saw it as the quintessential response.

The trio of friends was inseparable. They sat in Jane's tiny apartment and talked. Youth usually evaporates slowly, but for Jane Doe, it died that one day in September. AIDS had blasted the idealized future off her screen.

Her contracting HIV on the job had horrified those few nurses and doctors involved in her case at the hospital. Gerberding was upset. To be sure of her assertion, the doctor went back to the serum she'd saved from Jane Doe's initial participation in the health-care workers study that spring. Without notifying the labs about what she was looking for, she resubmitted it for testing. Again the results came back negative. Gerberding took a history from Jane Doe and asked about possible transmission of the disease through sexual contact or needle use. Jane

Doe had not engaged in risky behavior. It was clear that the nurse had been negative at the time she provided the study with her baseline specimen.

And there was no doubt she was now positive. Three weeks after she was given the information, Jane Doe flew to New York to tell her parents. She didn't know how she had lasted so long. On the slow plane ride home she felt she was packing a machete. When Jane Doe had called to say she was coming for a visit, she'd claimed she just had some extra time and money. Her parents didn't buy it. Her father suspected she was coming home to tell them she was getting married.

She arrived at night, when her mother already was asleep. Just after breakfast on an Indian summer morning, she told them. It was the hardest thing she ever had to do. She thought it made dying look easy. They were devastated, but they didn't blame her for choosing to work at the General, for knowingly working with AIDS patients, and they didn't tell her she should come home, which was just as well, because she wouldn't have. "What were they going to say," she said later. "'Leave the mecca? We can do better for you than in San Francisco?'" Both supportive, they were most concerned about what it was doing to their oldest child. Her father never worried about things until they happened. Her mother was the designated worrier of the family. She cried but was rational. She didn't say, "See, I told you so." She didn't claim, "Nobody listens to me." What she said was, "This is what happens in life."

They never had the luxury of thinking that perhaps the tests had been wrong. Jane Doe made it clear "This is it. There's no getting out of it." Her family kept her diagnosis quiet. It was nothing they would want whispered around their community. Sometimes old friends would tease, "Well, I don't know if I want you to come near me if you work with people with AIDS."

Over the weeks and months, Jane Doe worried about every rash and lymph node, every imagined symptom. One night, she and Jonathan appeared at the home of AIDS nurse Rita Fahrner, so concerned were they about Jane Doe's white tongue. She feared she had thrush (a white fungus that is often a sign of immunosuppression—people who don't have HIV disease also get thrush).

Fahrner shone a flashlight in Jane's opened mouth. She questioned her young friend until Jane remembered it wasn't thrush at all but the result of something she had eaten that night: feta cheese.

Jane Doe assumed, the way people do, that her employer, the city of

San Francisco, would take care of her. She assumed that any expenses she incurred would be paid by the city. And she assumed that with the exception of a few individuals the city need not know her real identity. She wanted to keep that information quiet. She didn't want her health insurance carrier to be informed because she wanted to keep her policy. She didn't want people to be afraid of her. She didn't want to risk being ostracized. She was too private a person to want her condition made public. Condolences, however well intentioned, could immobilize her. Discrimination, even in such a humanitarian city as San Francisco, could always happen. It never occurred to her that the city couldn't handle an anonymous nurse. It never occurred to her that the city's retirement system might doubt her claim or the veracity of what the doctors at the General confirmed.

In time, Jane Doe told a few more friends. The friend who was so frightened of AIDS she refused to dine in the Castro asked Jane Doe over the phone, "Do you know this nurse who got the AIDS virus?" Jane told her the truth. The friend brought an African dinner she'd made to Jane's apartment. When they were clearing the dishes, Jane advised her friend that she could use alcohol to clean her plates. "Don't insult me," said the friend, whose fear of AIDS had dissipated when she realized it now affected Jane Doe. Others were less understanding. Some told Jane that clearly, this was what God had meant for her. Others said, "God must really be impressed with you to throw such a big thing at you." One friend suggested that Jane did it to herself as a way of getting her life in order. Another allowed as how at least she'd always be skinny. "It's understandable to want a theory, to want a package wrapped up in a ribbon and put a neat bow on," Jane Doe said. "A lot of people did that. It's really human to do that, but it's kind of hard to be the recipient . . . . We walk around with this tremendous denial about mortality. It shows when people are confronted by it in a young person."

Some friends responded with what Jane called "harebrained theories and analysis." Without her seeking advice, many gave it. Some— especially those friends back East—told her that she should lead the life of a nun. Until then, Jane Doe had always been concerned with what other people thought. She no longer cared. Her sexuality had not been obliterated by the accident. There were safe means. When a friend asked her, "Why would you ever want to?" Part of her, the old part, saw herself as a young Catholic woman, a victim/martyr. Another part said, "Hell no!" So when the friend confronted her, Jane shot back, "I'll deal with my losses, but I am not going to create one more degree of loss than I need to." She was angrier still: "It's not enough that I've lost having a child. It's not enough that I've lost possibly fifty years of my life. It's not enough that I've lost peace of mind. I should take it even further? No way! This is a major loss, but don't make it bigger than it is."

She and her friend Jonathan became closer. And his family embraced Jane Doe, too. The relationship helped her through the early months. She didn't feel she was going through the crisis alone. And it helped her with the fight yet to come.

Only a few people at the hospital would ever learn who she was. Rumors abounded about what floor she worked on. The hospital's chief executive officer, Phillip Sowa, never knew her true identity. Jane Doe liked being anonymous at work, although she came to feel safe on the job only when there was someone on her shift who was informed—in case she wanted to freak out, which she didn't do.

Quirky hospital dramas gave her faith to go on.

One night two of her charges were AIDS patients. One, with toxoplasmosis, must have been a short-order cook in his heyday. Through the night, the patient howled: "Two cheeseburgers! One order of fries! Two cheeseburgers! One order of fries!" On and on. He wanted someone, anyone, to be with him. The nurses did what they could, soothing him when they had the time. If he learned a nurse's name, he'd call it incessantly.

Nearby was another AIDS patient, struggling with his fourth bout of PCP, the AIDS pneumonia. Nightmares were interrupting his sleep. Nightmares about then President Reagan. Disease and politics were entwined in his mind. Having been the designated speaker when the Presidential Commission on AIDS visited the hospital, he had reached out to shake hands with a commission member, only to have her refuse to shake.

That night, the patient roamed the ward, answering the telephone and other patients' lights.

In the morning, he learned that his mother died. Because of his debilitated state, he couldn't go to her funeral. The next night, his insomnia worsened. Meanwhile, the short-order cook blared his own American litany: "Two cheeseburgers! One order of fries!"

Reduced to small deeds in hospital corridors, the patient with the insomnia went to the patient yelling for burgers and fries and, at four in the morning, held his hand and calmed him. Without knowing it, he gave Jane Doe strength to move on.

If you can do it, she thought, I can do it. We're in this together.

She knew the short-order-cook patient and the patient with the insomnia were going to die. With her help, their deaths would be more comfortable. But for herself, she had hope. She had time. The General was one of the centers for AIDS drug tests. AZT could extend life by at least a few months, but other drugs, she reasoned, would come along soon.

War Declared

In a hospital conference room, Dr. Sande, the affable, gray-haired chief of medicine at San Francisco General, who had let Volberding build the AIDS program, gave the chiefs of services the news about Jane Doe. With this announcement, on October 2, 1987, the hospital began a debate about physician responsibility that would continue over years and across countries.

As Sande made the announcement, Dr. Lorraine Day, the hospital's chief of orthopedic surgery, saw her life pass before her. The mother of two boys, she had felt safe, at least until then. She had told her residents and interns they had nothing to worry about. Along with everyone else, Day had been relying on the experts at the hospital and at the federal Centers for Disease Control who, she recalled, told her it was "impossible" for her to contract the disease on the job.

As Sande spoke, only Day was critical, even hostile. She resented, she said, how he had "lied to me" and she resented "the cavalier way" she felt he presented the news. He was talking about a nurse who had

58

contracted a deadly disease while working at the hospital. The nurse was going to die at an early age. But in his low-key manner, Sande didn't speak about death and dying but about a nurse who "seroconverted."

"Sounds like she got religion," Day said. "Merle," she went on, "I'm under the impression this woman has a one-hundred-percent chance of getting AIDS. Am I right?"

"Yes," Sande replied.

"Then I understand that she has virtually a one-hundred-percent chance of dying of AIDS. Am I right?"

"Yes, you are right. But of course we don't say that publicly."

"Why?" Day asked in anger. "We must tell the public how fatal this disease is."

"We don't want to take away the hope of AIDS patients," he replied.

"Well, that is a false hope. I think anyone dying of the disease has a right to know that," Day said. (This account was provided by Day. Sande has no recollection of it, but he agrees that he would never say that the disease is 100 percent fatal.)

In a village lacking electricity, Lorraine Day would have stood out like red neon. At fifty, with her coiffed blond hair reaching to her shoulders, she could still earn a living modeling, as she had in her youth. She had a perfect nose, clear blue eyes, modest makeup and a gym-refined figure. Or she could become a TV anchor, as one feature writer suggested. But when she's described as having the look of a prom queen or a first-class stewardess, she bristles that those descriptions are degrading. "They make me sound like an airhead!" she complains, although no one who has ever met her would mistake her for that.

While northern California women tended toward earth tones, Day wore primary colors: strong yellows, blues and reds that set off her tanned good looks. Her clothes were southern California jazzy: scoop necks, skirts above the knee and thin high heels that went click-click down the halls. In fact, her clothes were functional. For years, she had to be in and out of the operating room many times each day. She needed scooped-necked tops, for example, that she could quickly slip in and out of. As for her high heels, they, too, she said were functional. They made her bad back feel better.

Her appearance only accentuated the differences between her and her colleagues. San Francisco is one of the last bastions of left-wing politics, where anyone who votes a moderate Democratic ticket is considered a conservative. In this most liberal of cities, the General is one of its most respected institutions. Many of the hospital's doctors were molded by the sixties.

Every spring, when the massive gay freedom parade wended its outrageous way through San Francisco with Dykes on Bikes, the San Francisco Gay Men's Chorus, moderate gay groups and those dressed only in leather jockstraps, the nurses from 5A, the General's AIDS ward, marched and received some of the loudest cheers.

Early in the epidemic, the General earned a national reputation for receptiveness to AIDS patients. And Volberding came to symbolize the goodness of a public institution responding to a feared epidemic. So many physicians were making pilgrimages to the hospital that Dr. Wofsy, one of the hospital's first AIDS doctors, designed a regularly scheduled program for visiting physicians (later funded by grants from the Bay Area's musicians Huey Lewis and the News). San Francisco General was an oasis in a dry plain of ignorance.

Yet in the midst of the epidemic, surrounded by these physicians and nurses emphasizing compassion, Day emerged. "No epidemic ever got under control with the use of compassion," she said. "They were doing nothing to stop the spread of the epidemic!" Her presence at the General was as incongruous as finding George Bush sojourning at a Vermont commune.

The hospital's doctors and nurses found her outrageous, embarrassing and wrong. Attempts were made to bring her down or throw her out. But Day was a smart, well-regarded surgeon, and she was tough and unyielding. She challenged the hospital's assumptions, mocking its liberal do-good policies. Hospital policy observed the regulations set down by the Centers for Disease Control, known as universal precautions. That included the wearing of gloves, masks and goggles when needed.

"Universal precautions in the operating room are a joke," Dr. Day fumed. "That's what we've been doing for fifty years! Gloves. Gowns. That was mainly for the patient," she said. A lot of it, she said, was only lip service. Telling surgeons to use universal precautions is "like saying 'If you're cold, why don't you just get dressed every day?' You've been getting dressed every day since you've been born. It's just so stupid. It just shows they don't have any idea what the problem is!"

Blood. A splatter in the eye. A spray into the nostril. Blood on the skin. A scalpel scrapes. A needle slips. Drill on bone and blood becomes airborne. Pools of blood form on operating-room floors. Surgeons, especially orthopedic surgeons, were awash in it. Trauma surgeons, unaware of their patient's HIV status, had begun wearing knee-high boots, two or three pairs of gloves, masks, goggles and protective aprons. In an era of new fears and little real discussion, Day became the only monologue in town.

At the chiefs of service meeting, Day made her first move. For her own protection and that of her staff, she said she was going to ask her nonemergency-surgery patients to be tested for AIDS. If a patient tested positive, she might provide an "alternative" to surgery. If, on the other hand, Day considered surgery essential, she and the operating room staff would be able to shield themselves with extra protective gear. Hospital policy opposed testing patients unless it was for the patients' benefit. The administration was reflecting AIDS patients' concerns that the results might cause them to lose their insurance, jobs or housing. (To satisfy state law on AIDS test results [only those involved in the patient's medical care could be informed] the General employs three full-time hospital workers to white out references to HIV status in medical records before they are sent to other hospitals or physicians.)

After speaking to the chiefs, Sande called together the hospital staff to confirm what had already become a widespread rumor—that a nurse at the General had acquired the AIDS virus on the job. His confirmation shocked many. In McGrath's lab, where researchers worked with live virus, the announcement was frightening and sobering. Researchers began to take extra precautions. So did nurses and physicians at the General. But Day's response was more aggressive.

Six days after the meeting in Sande's office, war was declared.

One of Day's patients, who had an ankle fracture from a motorcycle accident, refused to be tested for AIDS. He told the *San Francisco Chronicle* he'd been scheduled for surgery but that when he refused to be tested, the staff said he no longer required the surgery. Anonymous hospital sources chastised Day in print. "The hospital has some of the world's experts formulating infectious control procedures," one said. "It doesn't serve anyone well to have a single chief of service going off on her own."

Another anonymous source said that if patients are HIV positive, "they're probably going to get different treatment—which she [Day] will try to justify by all sorts of surgical arguments."

The *Chronicle* story added that, "No other San Francisco hospital contacted by the *Chronicle* has instituted a policy similar to Day's."

Ankle fractures can be treated by surgery or with casts. Most ankle fractures at the General are operated on. "Our patients may not come back," Day later explained. "They may live under a bridge. So we have a tendency to fix them in the operating room because then we know we've got them." In the case of the patient with the ankle fracture who refused to take the AIDS test, his fracture was in excellent alignment, in a proper cast, before Day had asked that he be tested. "He received excellent treatment," Day said. And he returned for follow-up care. No operation was necessary, she said, although she added that if he'd required one, she would have operated.

The hospital was dead set against her. Day knew she was alone. "All these men who had been at the committee meeting went off and hid under their desks," she complained. "They all lied about it. They spoke anonymously . . . and said we didn't agree to this, when they had.

"Then I thought, They're a bunch of wimps. They're about as gutless as you can imagine. I knew I was going to have to go it alone."

When other doctors told her not to request the test for every patient, Day objected. "Are you out of your minds? Don't you care about our lives? You know, this is craziness. People in the bureaucracy have compromised their principles so much that they don't even hear their conscience anymore."

Dislike, even hatred, for her snowballed through the hospital. At Ward 86, the AIDS outpatient unit, a sign with a child on it read PLEASE HUG ME. I HAVE AIDS. Scrawled below in pencil someone had written, GO AWAY LORRAINE DAY.

Meanwhile, Day was becoming famous in the medical community. She spoke for many scared surgeons awash in blood and for other physicians who felt that AIDS was being treated as a civil-rights issue rather than a medical one.

In an environment in which physicians tended to be collegial, Day was sometimes abrasive and often argumentative. "If you run a service you have to have some backbone," she complained.

She'd gone to medical school in the days when women were supposed to be helpmates, not peers. In the abstract, she seemed like the ideal feminist—driven, direct and successful in the macho-jock world of orthopedic surgery. She was also a UCSF associate professor of orthopedic surgery. But rarely did she emit sisterly vibes.

Before AIDS, her reputation as an excellent surgeon, loyal to her chief, was unblemished. Dr. Dick Fine, the hospital's onetime chief of staff and chair of the HIV policy committee, found her "an aggressive, intelligent, dedicated orthopedic surgeon," even though he couldn't stand her politics. During the antiwar years, she'd subtly suggested that Fine and friends were wasting their time in protest. When San Francisco State University students rebelled over Third World issues, Fine organized the medical support for protesters injured in clashes with police. He prevailed on some doctors and residents to list the demonstrators' extensive injuries and to write down the patients' exact words, to help the demonstrators when they went to court.

Over the years, Fine had lost none of his radicalism. In his hospital office he'd hung a whale mobile. A pin on the wall read WELCOME HOME STEPHEN BINGHAM, a reference to the leftist lawyer accused and acquitted of smuggling a gun to San Quentin prison radical George Jackson in 1971. The incident led to the deaths of six people. Although he now wore a Casio watch on his wrist, he sometimes sported a Minnie Mouse earring.

He knew he could never prevail upon Day, but Fine still admired her brand of success. As AIDS invaded the hospital, the two frequently disagreed over hospital policy. There was no longer any subtlety to their differences. And in the hospital at least, Day tended to be a minority of one. But numbers did not intimidate her. "In a couple of years I will be vindicated," she said. "They will hate me more because I was right."

"I am the leading spokesperson because I'm in the hotbed of AIDS. I have a reasonable interest in staying alive," she said. "I train interns and residents. I feel responsible for their lives."

Others might have campaigned with a modicum of diplomacy. They might have cajoled, strategized, compromised. That was never Day's style. She was only eleven when she realized that not everybody liked everybody else and that sometimes people compromised their principles because they wanted to be liked. "You had to make a decision whether you were more interested in being liked or standing on your principles."

Still, she was a normal girl of the 1950s. A very feminine child, she had "a pretty shop," a pretend store in her house with fake perfumes and decorative vases. In college, she majored in music, planning to teach piano to children. When she found she liked science, she switched to dental hygiene. Despite encouragement to become a dentist from her father, a minister high in the Seventh Day Adventist Church, she demurred. Women who became dentists and doctors, she felt, were "very masculine." She wanted to get married. The day after she graduated from college, she did.

Her first husband was in law school. Dutifully, Day joined the law wives' club. There, she learned how to play bridge and discuss detergents. She hated bridge and the idle life. At twenty-four, she enrolled in medical school. Her husband opposed it. They later divorced. She met her second husband, Dr. Larry Way, while she was in medical school and he was a young professor there. She paid her way through school working as a hygienist.

But few at the General knew about her background, and it probably wouldn't have made a difference anyway. Many gay nurses and others saw Day as a stick figure. Her platform, they were sure, rested on a scaffold of homophobia. But Day was more complex than that. Two of her four staff members were homosexual.

Too many experts in San Francisco were afraid to offend gays, she said. "The whole thing is politics," she declared. "If this had started out in the heterosexual community, the disease would be under control. Absolutely, because we would not have had a huge network of minority advocacy for this.

"For many years, the gays were discriminated against for all the wrong reasons. They are very upset about this and rightly so. So they wanted to have equal rights. All right. Unfortunately the sexual freedom they received finally and exploited in the bathhouses, which became death chambers, they didn't want to give up. They viewed it as their right to be an individual. Now they're very organized and they don't want to be trodden upon and they don't want to be put back in the closet. I can understand that . . . . Gay men have very strong interest in having their freedom and their rights and I don't say that that is wrong. They also have no children to raise and so preserving their rights is a major focus of their lives. The rest of the world doesn't feel as strongly about this . . .

"However, we've got two different things now. We've got gay rights to have proper jobs, housing and all that and we've got a deadly disease that can kill the world, and the two are being mixed up."

Day was challenging the General and the AIDS establishment. Some denounced her. Others were gunning for her.

I Don't Knuckle Under

The newspaper article about Dr. Day's plan to ask patients to be tested for AIDS before deciding on surgery started the battle that would rage not just at the General but throughout UCSF and beyond.

"In response to that article I got a call from the UCSF attorney," Day said. "I was in the operating room getting more exposure. He called me up in the operating room. He didn't say, 'Is any of this true?' He didn't say, 'What is this, can you tell me about it?' He said, 'If anybody sues you for anything in that article, you're not covered by malpractice.'"

Her story, the UCSF attorney, Joseph Cowan, said later, was accurate, as far as it went. He remembered the conversation well. He said he called her because he was returning her call.

When told she was performing surgery, he asked to leave a message. Hundreds of times in the course of his career, Cowan had telephoned surgeons. Never had he interrupted surgery. "You never go through to the operating room," he said. But Day's assistant insisted Cowan speak to her immediately. The call was put through. Cowan heard the clatter of medical instruments in the background. "I had this bizarre image come to mind of Dr. Day operating on someone's hip . . ."

She asked him about her liability, he recalled. If she tested a patient without his consent, she asked, would she be covered if the patient sued? Cowan told her that was a misdemeanor. He explained that if a civil action was brought against her by the patient and punitive damages were awarded, the university could not provide coverage. She responded, "Thank you very much. That's all I need to know."

Day angrily denies Cowan's account. "He's lying through his goddamn teeth!" she said. She claimed she would never test a patient for AIDS at the General without his consent and that the consent form had to be attached to the patient's tube of blood. "All that is crap," she declared. "I never asked him any of these questions. It never happened!"

Publicly, Day said, doctors at the General "are against my stand. Privately, many come to me and say, 'You can't imagine the support you have.' I cup my hand to my ear and say, 'Where are their voices?'"

"One reason other people aren't willing to speak out is because they see what's happened to me," she said. "I don't knuckle under . . . . They've been trying to shut me up all along by intimidating me, threatening me, threatening my job, all this crap. They thought I was just one person. They could take me by the neck, twist it and I'd stop. They didn't realize I have the support of virtually all fifteen thousand orthopedic surgeons in this country. I feel compelled to go to speak to them."

Suddenly she was being asked to talk to medical groups and reporters. And when producers from *Oprah Winfrey*, *Crossfire* and the network morning shows telephoned, she agreed to appear on their shows. Once, when she was to debate other General doctors on *Nightline*, a hospital PR woman refused to let the TV cameras tape her in the building. Only Day had to conduct her interview elsewhere. "I was sent outside like a bad little girl," she explained. She went to the administration and warned, "You better back off. This is crazy." Later, the PR tactic was recognized as a major blunder. To Day, it was just an example of the hospital trying to shut her up.

The hospital's PR staff regularly posted news stories about the General's doctors and nurses. When stories were published about Day, they were not tacked up. She had become an embarrassment.

The hospital recognized Day's right to free speech, but it didn't endorse what she was saying. "The patient's right to confidentiality,"

Day complained, "supercedes my right to stay alive. There's something wrong there.

"Never before has a doctor been forced to take care of patients who withhold important medical information from him" she said. She could only test a patient after he had given his permission. She wanted to know her patients' HIV status for her own safety and, she said, for the patients' benefit. If she operated on an HIV-positive patient, she said, she might shorten his life by seven or eight years. With an already depressed immune system, she argued, the patient, would be more likely to develop an infection following the operation.

For protection against HIV-positive patients, Day and her residents donned "space suits" when performing surgery with high-speed power instruments that created aerosols. Resembling motorcycle helmets, the space gear provided a clear plastic cover over the face. While tubes pumped oxygen in, cooling the air, the headgear made it difficult for surgeons to hear one another during an operation. For their attire, Day and residents often were ridiculed. "What planet are you going to land on today?" someone would shout as the residents and Day scrubbed for surgery.

More than anything else, the space suits symbolized doctors' fears of AIDS. "It was," Day said, "common-sense protection from the un- known and from potential hazards." The hospital was anxious to show that Day was by herself. "Space suits are a phenomenon peculiar to Lorraine," Dr. Gerberding said with a laugh. "To try and create a situation of zero risk by testing patients or using space suits or whatever your modus operandi, is just not possible. Our doctors are at risk. That's part of the price they pay for the privilege and professional respon- sibility," she explained. Gerberding believed that physicians couldn't have it both ways: "'I accept no risk and I want all the status, glory and money.'" She, too, considered it common sense to take precautions. "Who would want blood on their clothes? Urine in their eyes? It's simply a matter of avoiding someone else's body fluid." But the solution, she and the hospital contended, was to abide by universal precautions.

Both Gerberding and Day could have been accused of oversimplifica- tion. Gerberding spent most of her time organizing her study and analyzing its data. Day spent hers in the operating room.

As part of her campaign, Day went to talk to UC chancellor Dr. Julius Krevans "to tell him we are at great risk."

"These are sharp," she said, placing in his hand a surgical instrument that resembled a narrow-gauge knitting needle. She didn't break his skin with it but she did apply a little physical pressure. "These," she said, "can cut." And then she went on, "We get blood all over us all the time." She asked him to "put someone high up in the university in charge of AIDS safety and work with us. Get us together with the equipment companies . . ."

Then, she said, "I sort of got a little pat on the head. Nothing happened."

She had read a medical journal article about another virus found in aerosols in operating rooms, and she worried that blood-borne particles from HIV-positive patients might be tossed into the air by surgical power tools. She worried that they might be wafting through the operating room like smoke in a restaurant, to be inhaled by nurses and doctors. She wanted someone to check the operating-room air and to provide safer equipment.

The hospital, UCSF and the Centers for Disease Control discounted Day's fears of HIV aerosolization. If she were correct, they said, hundreds of surgeons would already have been felled by the disease.

Day was unswayed. She wrote a letter to the university saying she was not going to do any elective surgery on HIV-positive patients until the air in the operating room was checked. She'd continue to do all the emergency cases.

"If you persist," she was told by a UC official, "we will take out papers to have you replaced."

"Then they went to my chairman [of her department] and said, 'If you don't get this woman to rescind this letter, we're going to remove all of your funding from your entire department.'"

She felt the massive bureaucracy pressing down on her.

She continued to ask patients to be tested for AIDS. And she continued to do nonelective surgery even though no one was testing air in the operating room.

She also encouraged her residents to be tested for AIDS although she didn't insist on it. She objected to Jane Doe's anonymity. She felt patients should have the right to know if their nurse was HIV positive. Day had no idea where in the General Jane Doe worked. For her part, Jane Doe knew exactly where to find Day. Although the two had not met, Jane Doe knew what Day stood for. She believed that Day was a symbol of fear and anger against people with the virus.

Sometimes hospital employees hid the HIV test-requisition slips from Day. Other times they postponed giving the test results to the surgeon.

AIDS doctors had heard stories that Day was scheduling patients for surgery, only to cancel the surgery on learning they were HIV positive. Day called them "lying bastards running around saying these things about me."

Without informing her, the hospital's quality assurance committee investigated her surgical cases to see if she had denied care to HIV-positive patients. Day contended that if someone was HIV positive the doctor had the right to provide alternative treatment to elective surgery, for bunions or a hip replacement. But critics, such as Dr. Molly Cooke, head of the hospital's nascent ethics committee and Volberding's wife, argued that for a hip-replacement patient in a wheelchair, painkillers were no substitute for surgery. Cooke called Day's alternative-treatment concept a "grotesque euphemism."

In an odd way, Day's strong stance helped the calm, analytical Cooke understand the public's fears. "I didn't have to wait to get letters from people in Arkansas," she said. "I used her to anticipate arguments. I learned a lot from seeing how she thought about problems. I think she advanced the argument," although, Cooke said, "she's really difficult to deal with and she didn't play fair."

An internist, Cooke and most of the other General physicians were focusing on patient needs. Day, the surgeon, was considering the risk-benefit ratio and how an operation might put operating-room staff at risk. "There is very little evidence that surgeons are being infected," Cooke countered, although Day claimed to have a secret list of surgeons infected with HIV on the job. Cooke felt Day's equation "was not acceptable because the loss of benefit to the patient [seeking a hip replacement] seemed excessive in comparison to the reduction of risk to the physician," Cooke said, adding, "but it doesn't seem so to Lorraine."

Once, Day had refused to perform surgery on a dying AIDS patient with a broken neck. He had what she called "that Rock Hudson look," of someone ready to die. She estimated he had maybe three weeks to live. He'd broken his neck after driving his car over a bank in a failed suicide attempt. His internist insisted she operate. She told him he was out of his mind. "He wanted me to contaminate everyone in the operating room for this man." The operation, she contended, would have done the sick patient no good. "He probably would have died on the table because of his respiratory problems," she said. Instead, she put the patient in a halo traction, a metal device that screws into the skull, keeping a patient's spine rigid. He died three days later—of AIDS.

The quality assurance committee investigated all of Day's HIV-positive cases, focusing on those that were controversial. The committee could find nothing wrong with Day's handling of patients, although Dr. John Luce, then chief of staff and later head of the quality assurance committee, believed that "true consent" from patients asked to take the AIDS test "was not gained." He suspected that Day was holding the threat of no surgery over some of her patients. The lovers of some surgery patients had telephoned to complain, but none had been willing to come forward to make the case against Day. "I never failed to believe that there were things that went on," Luce said. "It was just that we couldn't prove it."

Day was constantly fighting the AIDS majority. In 1988, she campaigned for California Proposition 102, which would have required physicians to report to the state the names of all HIV-positive patients and those suspected of being HIV positive. (The state already requires doctors to report other contagious diseases such as smallpox.) If the measure has passed, many of the General's physicians were preparing to destroy files or otherwise commit civil disobedience rather than hand over names.

Day was fighting on numerous fronts. That summer, she became embroiled in a blood drive dispute. A flyer posted on a hospital bulletin board sought volunteers to donate blood in the city's gay Castro district. Credit for the blood was to be given to AIDS patients unable to pay for blood transfusions. The drive by an organization called Arm in Arm and another drive a few weeks later by the Harvey Milk Democratic Club were lesbian-sponsored.

Day thought a blood drive in a gay neighborhood was absurd. She wrote Irwin Memorial Blood Bank asking, "Are you aware this is going to be in an area where gay men cruise?" The blood bank, she contended, was risking the purity of the blood supply for political reasons.

In a compromise that pleased no one, the blood bank refused to send its mobile unit to the Castro, which had one of the highest densities of AIDS patients in the United States, offering instead to ferry blood donors in its minivan from the Castro to the blood bank headquarters, where the donations could be made.

Lenore Chinn, head of the Harvey Milk Democratic Club blood

drive, and Penni Kimmel, head of the Arm in Arm drive, appealed to medical-school officials to reign in Day. The women and their supporters also appealed to the city and hospitals for backing.

Local AIDS doctors and politicians, including then Mayor Art Agnos, wrote the blood bank urging it to continue to collect blood through the lesbian programs in the Castro. San Francisco's gays were educated about AIDS, they said. And lesbians' blood was safer than that of heterosexual women. The drive also was open to men. They were to be screened by the lesbian groups and by Irwin Memorial nurses.

Again, Day was out there by herself. But she believed that many gay men were suffering "from an addiction, like cocaine or alcohol that they know can kill them and they continue to do it. They say [being gay] is genetic. To have a thousand sexual partners a year? There is no chromosome for that."

"If I see things happening that shouldn't be happening and I do nothing, I am contributing to that problem," she explained. *The Sentinel*, a gay paper in San Francisco, was not swayed. Its editorial accused Day of trying "to fan the flames of fear and bigotry by attesting that the drive would in some way endanger the safety of the blood supply."

Before the summer was over, Irwin Memorial acquiesced. By fall, the lesbian groups were back in the Castro, with the blood bank's mobile unit. For her part in the fight, Lenore Chinn, organizer of the Harvey Milk blood drive, was selected by the mayor to sit on the Human Rights Commission.

We Are All Jane Doe

Jane Doe never considered suing the hospital or the city for her injury. She hadn't even thought about finding a lawyer until urged to by friends. She just wanted to be reimbursed for her medical expenses— early visits to the doctor, checkups and psychological counseling as a result of the diagnosis. She expected the city to pick up future medical costs. Given the stigma attached to AIDS, she sought relative anonymity so that her employer, coworkers, future employer or landlord need not know. But the city wanted her to hand over her name, purely for administrative purposes.

In other communities, the concern might not have been for Jane Doe so much as for patient safety. But in San Francisco, an atoll of liberalism, that was barely an issue. If everyone who was HIV positive had to quit the General, the hospital could not function. Occasionally Dr. Day complained that she didn't know where Jane Doe worked, but in time she narrowed her focus, contending that a patient having an invasive procedure done had the right to know if his doctor was HIV positive, just as she argued that a doctor should have the same right to know about a patient's infectious status. But as usual, Day was out there by herself. More common was the attitude of Dr. Dick Fine, who argued that a patient was "more likely to be hit by an asteroid," than contract AIDS from a nurse or doctor. "Unfortunately," explained Dr. Molly Cooke, "there are many aspects of being a patient that pose much more risk." A patient is more likely to have the wrong limb amputated, the wrong medication prescribed or have his physician confuse him with another patient. In fact, there had never been a reported case of a patient being infected by his doctor or nurse anywhere in the United States. (The case of dentist David Acer infecting Kimberly Bergalis and four other patients was not yet known. Even now, there still are no reported cases of doctors or nurses infecting patients, while there are several dozen cases of patients infecting doctors and nurses.)

Jane Doe's right to remain anonymous was still an issue. She was willing to inform a few people in city government, only a few. But the city retirement board felt Jane Doe's claim should be processed like any other. Jane Doe would have to let them investigate her work history, her social life, specifically her sex life. Bureaucrats would reserve the right to inform whomever they felt they had to inform if she were going to be paid.

When Jane Doe's attorney, Patricia Hastings, called the city to negotiate on Jane Doe's behalf, she expected no problems. She had previously worked for the retirement board. But when she called them about Jane Doe, she was told they couldn't discuss the case because the city had no way of knowing if Hastings really represented the injured employee. Despite the newspaper accounts about Jane Doe, TV stories and declarations from doctors and administrators at San Francisco General, the city claimed not to know if such a nurse existed. And if she existed, officials said, how were they to know she was employed by the city and county of San Francisco?

Reasonable questions, they were answered almost immediately by the hospital, the doctor in charge of the health-care workers study, and the nurses' union, which agreed to act as liaison between Jane Doe and the city. But the retirement board, which doled out workers' compensation, would not be satisfied.

Jane Doe and attorney Hastings came to believe the city's reluctance to negotiate was all about money. It was not inconsistent with an explanation given by the general manager of the Employees Retirement

System, the crusty Clare Murphy, who said that if she agreed to Jane Doe's anonymity request, "I could be forced to open the faucet which I could never close and be accountable for every unit of water that went through it."

There would be other cases of workers contracting the AIDS virus on the job, but none would be as well documented as the case of Jane Doe. She had donated blood frequently over the years, so there existed a trail of proof that she had been HIV negative. The very month she began working at San Francisco General, she had donated blood. Two months before the needle-stick, Jane Doe participated in the San Francisco General AIDS health-care workers study, and she tested negative. Tests were conducted less than a month after the needle-stick and then six days later. The difference between them showed clearly that a seroconversion was occurring. (The antigen test measured proteins specific to the virus. The antibody test measured the body's reaction to the presence of the virus.) Dr. Julie Gerberding, head of the health-care workers study, concluded that early on, when the virus was circulating in Jane Doe's body, the antigen test was positive. Then as Jane Doe's body began its immune response, the antigens cleared out of the bloodstream. The antigen test became negative while the antibody test turned positive. One of the world's leading authorities on the occupational AIDS infection, Gerberding called Jane Doe's case "absolutely classic for occupational infection."

Before agreeing to take the case, attorney Hastings had grilled Jane Doe. A lesbian with pinprick humor, Hastings wanted to be "damn sure there were no holes in this case because I knew it was precedent setting and I wanted the most righteous case in the world . . . . I made sure I could put her up against the Virgin Mary."

Hastings knew that ordinarily a worker relinquishes his privacy when he files a workers' compensation claim. But the attorney expected that in the case of Jane Doe, the city would show compassion. She did not expect a showdown.

Traditionally nurses have been a docile lot, or at least they've been perceived that way. Jane Doe and her attorney were not. "She would have had to be a kamikaze nurse from hell trying to commit suicide by injecting herself with HIV in order for this incident not to be compensable," Hastings said.

San Francisco General, its doctors, nurses and administrator had shown understanding and sympathy, even though most didn't know who Jane Doe was or even where in the hospital she worked. The mayor's office had expressed concern. But the city retirement board would not be moved.

Jane Doe continued on the job, believing in the goodwill of the hospital and the city of San Francisco. "You work for an organization, you get hurt, they take care of you," she said. She wasn't in a litigious mood. In the beginning, at least, she was just coping. Getting to work each day. Going home. Just trying to get by. She let her pro bono attorney Hastings, whom she would describe as "a mega-softie under the armor," handle the city.

Following early negotiations between her union and the city's retirement board, the young nurse was told to submit medical claims along with a code number. Using her grandmother's date of birth, she whited out her name on the medical bills, submitted them and waited. The General's director of nursing, Brenda Lauer, offered to act as liaison. Lauer was one of the few who knew who Jane Doe really was. But when the bills were submitted, Lauer was told that the code number was insufficient. The city would not pay a claimant unless her name was known. That Gerberding, too, could vouch for her employment and existence, was not persuasive. Gerberding and others from the hospital were seen as partisan.

Drawn-out negotiations were begun. At one point, Hastings suggested Jane Doe's file be locked in a box at the retirement board office. Officials balked. They said senior people could not waste time looking after a locked box. ("What the hell is that senior executive going to do?" Jane Doe asked, "stare at the filing cabinet from nine to five?")

The retirement board suggested Jane Doe file the claim as stress-induced/work-related ailment. "I really needed that on my record . . . psychologically impaired," said Jane Doe.

The city attorney's office and the retirement board suggested Jane Doe submit her claim as a finger injury, using her real name. It was a suggestion the retirement board pushed and pushed. "That was the best that all these minds could come up with," Jane Doe marveled. "It's the stupidest solution," she said, imagining putting in bills for "a little AZT for my index finger."

The city's inability to accommodate Jane Doe seemed rooted in history. Its that's-how-things-are-done attitude infuriated her. A new policy, she felt, would be seen as cumbersome and inconvenient. Every little request seemed to be such a disruption for the bureaucrats. "Like, this isn't disruptive to my life?" Jane Doe asked.

Despite her friends, her lover, her family, more and more she was feeling alone with the pain in her head. Sometimes she expected others to make it better. She considered locating other HIV-positive women, who might make her feel less alone. In San Francisco, a woman with the HIV virus didn't have the same support that gay men had. With initial misgivings, she joined a support group of women with HIV disease, although she knew no one else in the San Francisco group would have contracted the disease from a needle-stick.

There Jane Doe found twelve "vibrant, healthy, intelligent women." The group shocked her. One was a beautiful blond with flowing hair. Jane Doe's first reaction was to think that so gorgeous a woman couldn't possibly be HIV positive. "I'm not proud of these feelings," she said, but she had believed the myth that nothing bad happened to beautiful people. Intellectually she knew she wasn't the only person walking around with the pain. But there was no substitute for seeing, talking, hugging, laughing and crying with others. They shared so much. So much only they thought about. Each month when they got their periods, they thought that their blood could be deadly.

How each woman had become infected (IV drug use, sexual transmission, blood transfusions and Jane Doe's sole needle-stick) made no difference when it came to understanding one another's pain. They commiserated, talking about the stigma and the loss. When she was with her support group, Jane Doe didn't have to deal with the smiling faces: "You just have to keep a positive attitude," or "Look at the bright side."

Like a lot of other HIV-positive people, Jane Doe started attending to how she lived. She began consuming vast amounts of vitamin C, vitamin E, vitamin B complex, iron and multivitamins. She signed up to participate in an AIDS study of Chinese herbal medicines. She regularly consumed a combination of herbs from deer antlers, ginseng, tortoiseshell, peony, citrus, cardamom and licorice. She cut down on the Cheese Doodles and Big Macs, on sugar, fats, red meat and caffeine. She went to exercise class several times a week and started spending a lot more time outdoors.

Although she showed no symptoms of the disease, her awareness of her body became acute. When in the company of other HIV-positive people, they talked about doctor visits, pills, aches and little chills. The virus seemed to have accelerated the aging process. She was only twenty-six. Other twenty-six-year-olds, unencumbered with HIV, weren't thinking the way she was. With HIV came some of the wisdom usually reserved for the old who've lived through or seen friends live through hard times.

When she was visiting family in a New York suburb, Jane Doe often forgot about AIDS, forgot about herself. AIDS didn't seem to be so prominent in the suburban mind the way it was in San Francisco. And the East was where she'd grown up, where she'd lived before the needle-stick. Even in San Francisco, Jane Doe's pain was episodic. Much of the time her attention was diverted toward fighting the city.

In the summer of 1988, she took leave from her job at the hospital and vacationed in Europe. She'd given up her apartment, because she and her friend Jonathan were going to be moving in together. When she returned to the city her relationship was breaking up; she had no apartment and no money; and an HIV-positive friend from work, the rock of her life, was showing the symptoms of AIDS. Next, she learned no progress had been made with the city. She started spending spare hours lying in bed in the dark. She called Regina, her old friend from Minnesota, who had come out when Jane Doe was diagnosed. Jane Doe's situation frightened Regina. Without consulting Jane Doe, Regina made the next move. Sitting at a word processor in the law library where she studied, the friend composed a letter to Randy Shilts, author of the book *And the Band Played On* and a top *San Francisco Chronicle* reporter covering AIDS. In the letter, Regina described Jane Doe's dilemma. Jane Doe recognized the city of San Francisco was saturated with HIV so that even if she chose to bring her case to the press, it might not be of real interest. Regina asked if Shilts thought it newsworthy.

Randy Shilts gave the letter to *Chronicle* reporter Elaine Herscher, who telephoned Regina to say the newspaper wanted the story. Her friend then called Jane Doe and confessed. Relieved, Jane Doe felt that Regina had kicked open another door. It had always been hard for Jane Doe to plead for herself. She didn't like saying she was being treated unfairly because "in the grand scheme of things what I was going through was so minimal."

Under the headline NO BENEFITS YET FOR AIDS INFECTED NURSE, published on March 13, 1989, the story described Jane Doe's "terrible trauma," and the fact that for nineteen months the city had refused to reimburse her for the four thousand dollars she had incurred in medical expenses. In a weak reply, city officials claimed they could not pay Jane Doe under confidentiality conditions required by law. "I believe the claim should be paid as soon as we have the ability to insure that the employee is an employee of the city and county," said Murphy, head of the retirement system. Her comment made it clear that a year and a half of negotiations had led nowhere.

Mayor Art Agnos's office tried to pressure Murphy, too. If she'd been a mayoral appointee, "it would have been fixed in fifteen seconds," said Larry Bush, Agnos's speechwriter and liaison to the gay community. Murphy had been appointed by a seven-member board of which Agnos appointed only two members. In a meeting called by the mayor's office, Murphy claimed California law would not permit her to lower the number of persons needing to be informed.

But Bush had written the law for Agnos on the consent and confidentiality of AIDS antibody results. The law limited who could legally reveal HIV status. And it made no provisions for an administrator to tell a third party, as Murphy insisted she must.

That spring, 48 Hours called attorney Hastings requesting that Jane Doe appear. In darkened cameo, Jane Doe spoke on camera about understaffing and accidents at the hospital (which the show used) and workers' comp (which it didn't).

News of Jane Doe's plight angered doctors and nurses at the General. The department of medicine offered her a no-interest loan of ten thousand dollars to hold her over, the money coming from concerned physicians such as Dr. Dick Fine, who had organized the fund. Through their unions, Service Employees International Union locals 790 and 250, San Francisco General employees called a dramatic press conference at which some thirty nurses and doctors appeared wearing Jane Doe name tags. In a gutsy speech, Gerberding said that by its inaction, the city was "sending a very clear message to us—you have to come and work and take the risk but we will not back you up and protect your confidentiality." She added, "We are all Jane Doe." Sasha Levine, one of the nurses most active in Jane Doe's behalf, said that if an agreement was not signed within a month, hospital workers would no longer perform risky medical procedures.

Startling Results

Nearly every morning before going to her lab at San Francisco General, Isabelle Gaston scrambled downstairs to confer with her gay neighbor, Chris Adams.

They sat on the back porch looking out on an apricot tree and Chris's herb-and-vegetable garden and talked AIDS. He taught Isabelle about AIDS politics—a free-lancer, he sometimes wrote about AIDS—and she taught him about the science. He cut out articles from the *New York Times* about AIDS activism. She brought him scientific journals that explained the disease.

Only a few years out of Barnard, Isabelle was a researcher in McGrath's lab. Some days her words tumbled out at great speed, as she told Chris about McGrath's theory that macrophages were the reservoir of HIV infection, with secondary loss of T cells.

Always eager to tell her friend of the experiment she'd done the night before, Isabelle would explain its significance. Chris already had ARC (AIDS-related complex), the precursor to full-blown AIDS. Having lived in the AIDS world for some time, Chris had seen plenty of hot prospects fail to pan out. So even when Isabelle was sharing her news, he viewed it "with a jaundiced eye," although he didn't say so. For her part, Isabelle was hopeful, but she didn't want to set herself and Chris up for a grotesque disappointment so she never said, "If you can hold on just a little longer, there might be a cure." But she thought it.

Some mornings she was so overwhelmed by Q's miraculous effect in the petri dish that she couldn't wait to talk to Chris. Even though she was living with her boyfriend, Chris was always the first to know.

At the lab, she felt she wasn't working hard enough. Sometimes she judged others harshly for not working hard enough either.

From 1985 until she went to McGrath's lab two years later, Isabelle had analyzed the blood of children with AIDS in the lab of retrovirologist Dr. Jay Levy. Even though she worked and lived in San Francisco, she knew no one with AIDS. Wanting to befriend people with AIDS, she trained to become a Shanti emotional support volunteer, spending her time off from work caring for one AIDS patient and helping the lover of another.

When she and her boyfriend moved to an apartment in the Haight Ashbury, Isabelle suddenly found herself surrounded by the AIDS community. Above her lived a women who offered massages to weakened, aching AIDS patients. Below lived three HIV-positive gay men. Chris Adams became one of Isabelle's closest friends.

The woman who had known no one with AIDS had become enveloped by it. Sometimes just going home to her apartment was painful. She couldn't help but see the steady stream of gay men visiting the masseuse upstairs. But it was also inspiring to be living near others working on AIDS.

Instead of going mountain biking with her boyfriend on some weekends, she returned to the lab. Some nights she wanted to check on her macrophages or set up new experiments. Because the building in which she worked was hidden from the street and its nighttime hallways were always darkened, she had Chris accompany her in her white Volkswagen Rabbit.

Lab science was a mélange of logic, art and cooking, Isabelle thought. What seemed like a relatively simple experiment to an outsider involved hundreds of other, more complicated experiments. McGrath had to establish how long a macrophage needed to be infected before adding the

Q. How long should Q be mixed with the sticky macrophages before it was washed out or before the cells were tested?

Using normal donor blood from Stanford Blood Bank, Isabelle isolated the macrophages and infected them with the virus she kept frozen in jars at minus-seventy degrees. After two weeks, she treated half of the infected macrophages with Q, at four different levels of Q concentration. Five days later, she measured the HIV proteins remaining in the cells. In the beginning, McGrath had planned to blitz macrophages, killing them all. Q did just that. Over time, however, he and Isabelle experimented with lower doses of Q.

Under McGrath's direction, Isabelle continued the daily tests. She admired him for his thinking—and his willingness to test an Eastern medicinal herb and his belief that Q should be thought of as a chemotherapeutic agent. He was, she thought, an iconoclast striving not to be a pariah.

By late spring of 1988, the Gaston-McGrath experiments were seeing startling results. Early one morning, Isabelle completed a large toxicity study that demonstrated that Q was minimally toxic on healthy, uninfected cells. Her finding would be meaningful only if Q was having an effect on the diseased cells. By that afternoon, Isabelle had amazing computerized results: in infected cells treated with Q, there occurred a 90 to 95 percent reduction of the AIDS virus. Isabelle was ecstatic.

McGrath could rarely sit still for her to copy the results into a more legible form. On this day, the anxious McGrath sped down the hallway, colliding with his excited researcher. The implications of their work were almost too amazing to imagine. In the petri dish, Q did what no other drug could do: it killed off diseased macrophages while leaving healthy cells alone.

Over and over again, Isabelle put on her latex gloves and conducted her experiments. And over and over, the results were clear, dramatic. They even shocked McGrath, who had no idea how a drug could possibly work so well. When the results were made public, news accounts were effusive. The *Village Voice* declared that, "This just might be the penicillin of AIDS."

Although their lab work didn't show it, McGrath quietly hoped that once Q killed the infected macrophages in humans, their depleted T4 cells, the critically important infection-fighting cells, would increase.

While Isabelle was conducting the experiments in the closet-size biohazard-containment room, McGrath's partner, Dr. Jeffrey Lifson, was reproducing them at Genelabs, a private biotechnology firm in Redwood City, a half-hour drive from the hospital. Lifson's results meant that McGrath's were less likely to be artifacts, artificial results caused by humans or other extraneous factors. While Gaston and McGrath studied Q's effect on macrophages, Genelabs examined Q's effect on T cells.

The partnership of Lifson and McGrath worked well. A born salesman, the gung-ho McGrath knew how to package his ideas to appeal for research grants. Lifson always had his foot firmly planted on the brakes. But both men became believers in Q, and together they swallowed their fears, boldly convincing Genelabs' board of directors that Q was worth pursuing. Based on two years of test-tube studies, Genelabs changed its focus from biotechnology to become a full-blown pharmaceutical development company. With the financial assistance of Sandoz Pharmaceuticals, it poured millions of dollars into research on Q.

Lifson and McGrath were lab scientists. They were neither businessmen nor as McGrath put it, "scale-up mavens." They had no background to draw from to know how to move from working with minuscule experiments to massive ones. "When you start out with giant vats of roots and having to purify a protein in FDA-approved fashion in an FDA-facility, you're talking a nightmare," McGrath said. No one at Genelabs had ever developed a drug before. The company had to figure out how to obtain the plant material from China, how to purify it, who to hire to do the development work. Because federal regulations require that research facilities be separated from drug development facilities, Genelabs had to build a new structure to accommodate the production of Q.

Animal toxicity studies were conducted in the United States and England. (McGrath is loath to name the species used out of concern that animal-rights activists would protest—even on such vital work as AIDS drugs research.) In most such FDA-approved studies, animals are given a daily dose of the drug over long periods of time. Scientists then test for toxins in each animal. But for Q such a procedure would have been absurd. If given every day over a long period of time, the experimental animals would either develop an immune response or a serious allergic reaction. If traditional methods were followed, Q would never be approved. McGrath and Lifson wanted Q developed like a chemotherapeutic. If it was to be given to humans, they believed it should be given intensively, a handful of times, to produce the greatest benefit.

McGrath and Lifson wanted to infuse the animals intermittently. But because their plans differed from the federal norm, they ran into difficulty with the FDA.

By 1989, Genelabs was producing Q for lab use, which they named GLQ223 (the GL stood for Genelabs). By then, Isabelle's Shanti AIDS client had died. Hurting over his death, she withdrew from her volunteer activities. But she continued to infuse her lab work with emotion, always thinking of her pal Chris and of his sick friends who had become her friends as well. Meanwhile, Chris was in a holding pattern. For several years, his T cell count remained relatively constant. If it dipped below a certain level, he thought he would try Q.

1989 TO THE PRESENT

In the Trenches

By the spring of 1989, AIDS had become pervasive at San Francisco General and its care was institutionalized. Every day one or two hospital workers called the hospital's innovative needle-stick hotline. Some had serious exposures. Others, including janitors and gardeners, had brushed up against needles of unknown origin.

What began as a calling for a few had become the daily work of everyone at the General. Doctors and nurses with no great interest in AIDS now were touched by it. HIV-positive patients were in every ward. Often they came with ailments unrelated to the virus.

Nowhere was the meeting between patients and staff more dramatic than in the emergency room. Hordes of patients and their relatives constantly were clamoring for instant care. Nurses and physicians responded by leaping into fast forward, even though their speed placed them in greater jeopardy.

But the wildness of the moment, the absurdity of humanity, the chaos of care gave the staff reason to remain even on days when they felt unappreciated.

Many of the ER patients acquired the virus through shared needles. Some of them used offensive language and self-destructive behavior while exhibiting little gratitude. Others were garden-variety alcoholics like Mr. Comstock.

"What hurts Mr. Comstock?"

The nose is bloodied, the face red raw, the hair matted and sun bleached. Through a drunken haze, he focused on the triage nurse in ER, familiar surroundings.

"My right leg."

"Your right leg always hurts," she said. Mr. Comstock was known on the ward as a frequent flyer.

"He's here for his nose," the paramedic intervened. Picked up where he lived, in Golden Gate Park, the patient had been knocked unconscious by someone wielding a skateboard.

It was the fourth time his nose has been broken. Other times he'd had other reasons to come, such as having lice and needing a shower.

"I'm not taking a shower" he said, even though no one had suggested it this time.

"He also said he has AIDS," the paramedic added.

"May I take a look at your nose?" a resident inquired.

"No!"

"We need to help you, sir." The doctor examined it anyway, pronouncing the nose "smooshed."

"Your nose is going to be fine," the doctor reassured, adding, "as fine as it was to start with."

Stretched out on a gurney in the ER hallway, Mr. Comstock did not want to cooperate.

"Don't move, sir," the young doctor advised, trying to put an IV line in place. From the catheter, blood dripped out, onto the doctor's gloved hand. Blood was taken for analysis and placed in four tubes. Because he was an alcoholic and probably dehydrated, Mr. Comstock was given fluids intravenously.

Everywhere there were subtle risks to health-care workers. The young doctor peeled off his gloves and picked up the four test tubes he'd filled with Mr. Comstock's blood. The rubber stopper for each tube had a pin-size opening used to break the vacuum and to allow the blood to be poured in, large enough for blood to seep out.

"It's no different than being a medic in a war," said a male nurse with the task of calming Mr. Comstock. "It's like playing Russian roulette. . . . People need medical service, so you weigh the risks."

Each nurse had made a decision about what he or she was willing to do.

Nurse Marley Gevanthor began considering her own safety five years earlier when she was pregnant with her first child. Occasionally she'd forget, pull off her glove and use her left index finger, her "peripheral eye," to find a vein. And often enough a doctor would scold, "Put your gloves on Marley, you've got a family."

Mr. Comstock was wheeled into the observation ward to sober up. Nurse Gevanthor cared for him and for Mr. Wall, another homeless alcoholic patient trying to postpone his departure. Gevanthor had already told him to polish off his dinner and leave. When she dipped into Mr. Wall's bag to retrieve his black jockey shorts, out spilled chunks of Iceberg lettuce, his evening's salad. In recent years the hospital had become a way station for people without resources. Alerted by do-good bystanders, the paramedics pried drunks and drug users off city streets, dumping them on the ER. Only the day before, Mrs. Rodriguez, a regular, was brought in three times within twenty-four hours, always with the same diagnosis: alcoholism. A street person, her final visit of the day came after she'd fallen flat on the street, in the middle of the city's Cinco de Mayo parade.

As Mr. Comstock came to, he grew nastier, bickering with Mr. Wall, a hallway roamer in hospital gown, wide open in the back.

The nastiness caused Nurse Gevanthor to become less enthusiastic. When patients flailed about, bit, scratched and kicked, she'd either call security and have them placed in four-point restraints or she would tell the doctor she couldn't start the IV or draw the blood. Her three- and four-year-old daughters came first. Yet there probably was no one on the ward better at starting IVs than the experienced Gevanthor. The doctors, many of whom were interns, were not yet used to dealing with junkies. She'd grown accustomed to putting a tourniquet on a patient and finding veins hard as tree branches. When dealing with IV drug users, Gevanthor easily drew blood from the groin rather than from an arm with no visible veins. That's what she had been doing on a gunshot patient one night, when a young, excitable doctor pushed his chest into her shoulder, shoving Gevanthor's needle into her hand. She didn't panic, but she did think God! Get this off me! And she had immediately rushed to the sink to wash blood from her hand. She had nabbed a red-top test tube full of the patient's blood to have it tested for HIV status. If she had been infected, her test results might not show it for several years. A negative result from the patient, while not conclusive, would make her feel better. But when she brought the tube to the AIDS health-care workers study office, Gevanthor was told that the blood could not be tested without the consent of the patient. The patient refused to be tested. Gevanthor thought it wasn't fair. "It's their rights versus mine. Mine are just as important or are more important." She'd been tested twice since then with negative results both times.

Sometimes when Gevanthor was transporting a test tube full of HIV-positive blood she felt she was carrying explosives. And sometimes when she walked out of the trauma room, she'd glance back at the blood-red rivulets on the operating room floor from an AIDS patient and she thought it was like exiting "a huge toxic waste dump. It looks just the same as everyone else's blood, but it's eating away at the patient." Times like that, Gevanthor wondered what she was doing there.

A young, angry patient was dropped off at the ER. "Ro-chelle did this!" he said as if her identity was known to mankind. "She came at me with a big-ass long thick knife and I thought it was a punch." He jabbered like a talk-show host. Ro-chelle, he announced, "was tweaking," coming off a drug high. He thought he could handle her. "I bench press two hundred twenty-five pounds every day," he said.

"Relax," said the male nurse in gloves and goggles, struggling to put the IV in. Blood from the wounds in the patient's abdomen was spilling out onto the sheet and down the gurney. Still the patient jerked about like a just-caught fish bouncing on the deck of a wooden boat. "My people are going to blow Ro-chelle's house up tonight."

"Please call your people off. That will only give us more business," said the good-humored nurse.

Meanwhile, the doctor tried to determine the depth of the wound, probing with round-edged instruments.

"Let me do it," the patient said, exhibiting muscle. "I said let me do it, man!"

A call went out for security.

The doctor needed to probe some more to find out where the knife went. "This is called 'Save your life now,'" the nurse explained. Next, he handed the difficult patient a urine sample bottle and asked him to donate.

"I can't do it. I'm not going to strain myself, man." The nurse needed a urine sample to check for blood.

"We just want to help you out," said an apple-cheeked doctor. The patient examined the wide-necked bottle with skepticism.

"One size fits all," they explained. His arms flailed about. He could be putting the staff at risk. He turned, tried to reach for various instruments. When the nurse attempted to insert a needle, he responded like a man under attack.

"You've got to chill out, guy," the nurse advised.

When the doctor tried to draw blood, the patient grabbed his name tag with the warning, "I'm going to come back looking for you."

It could all have been bravado, brought on by a life of deprivation or by a night of crack. Or it could have been serious. In addition to worrying about a return visit, the immediate risk was that through his gyrations, the patient could knock a needle into a nurse or doctor, dumping his blood on them.

Wheeled into the hallway, the patient continued his diatribe. Someone, he said, had called an ambulance for him but "It took too damn long. This hospital ain't shit. I betcha if I'd been on the avenues, they would have been there in three minutes. My homeboy had to drive me here. You all ain't no goddamn good." He continued flopping around the gurney, comparing the amount of blood puddled on his sheet with that of a gunshot patient nearby. And he offered pseudomedical advice until one of the doctors observed, "It's amazing how many doctors come in with stab wounds." Without humor, they couldn't function.

It's in the ER that weirdos are exposed to the culture of normalcy, however chaotic it is. Nurse Toni Maines, an earth mother with a don't-mess-with-me attitude, recalled the patient who shot peanut butter into his veins. She remembered the time the San Francisco Police Department phoned to say they'd found a penis in front of city hall, in case someone came in missing one. The night before a patient had come in with what nurses described as "rings in interesting places." But perhaps the most absurd patient was the one paramedics refused to tell her about. They insisted she inquire. While the patient was writhing on the gurney, Maines quizzed him.

"Sir, what's wrong?"

"My stomach."

"How long has your belly been in pain?"

"Since this morning. I know exactly what it is," he said, whereupon nurse Maines was shown Exhibit A, a Zip-Loc bag containing two bald Barbie doll heads.

"I eat these," he said. Another nurse explained that the patient enjoyed the eating and excreting of the objects.

X rays that later became popular in the medical underground, showed six other bald Barbie heads obstructing the man's bowels.

Another time, Maines recalled, a patient came in complaining because he'd pinned his penis to the skin of his abdomen and was unable to urinate. He had holes in his urethra. A few nights later, when Maines was moonlighting at another hospital, the same patient showed up, pinned again. Maines's comment to him: "You, man, are stupid!"

"There are a lot of weirdos out there," Manes said, "And we know every one of them."

At the front desk, a man brought in by ambulance was leaning in toward the triage nurse, as if to confide. Each time he slanted in toward her, he tried to nip her breasts. She pulled back, unfazed.

While one patient yelled at passersby, a hit-and-run victim was wheeled into the next trauma room. The paramedics warned that the man was high on PCP. The ER reserves a room for people coming off drugs. On the ceiling, someone had scrawled Nancy Reagan's motto: JUST SAY NO.

Another patient, familiar to the staff, rested on another gurney. In one of his periodic suicide attempts, he'd taken an overdose of his asthma medicine. Last time he had tried to kill himself it was because he thought he had AIDS. He didn't. A Mariel boat person, he had walked across the United States and had been treated in emergency rooms all across the country.

A short, squat, Spanish-speaking woman arrived with her family. She was wrapped in a yellow-and-white striped blanket and was wearing a beige wool beanie. For every question raised by the triage nurse: "How old is she?" or "What's wrong with her?" the family caucused before arriving at an answer.

At other hospitals, she might have been seen soon after she arrived. One nurse told another that "the patient is like a million years old." But the stab wounds, the gunshot victims, and out-of-control patients had to come first. In a febrile state, the old woman was placed in "the gurney garage," where patients rest while waiting to see a physician.

A young black woman made a dramatic entrance: "Let me see my momma!" she hollered.

"She's fine," the triage nurse advised. Having come in with chest pains, the mother had remained at the hospital for blood tests.

Quietly the nurse observed that despite the appearance of high drama, there were no tears.

Paramedics came in with another man picked up off the street. Wearing black lace stockings under his jeans and women's flats, the androgynous patient was described as an IV speed user and slightly paranoid. He told the nurse he'd come in because he wanted an HIV test. No tests were done at night, she told him. Then she ran down the list of questions.

"Why are you here?"

"I'm tired."

She looked at him quizzically, so he filled in the blanks. "I don't drink or eat for three days."

"Anything hurt?"

"Everything."

He was sentenced to the gurney garage.

Two organ-donor nurses wandered by in search of a liver. They were there to pick up the organ for an operation at another hospital.

"Volunteer to the front desk. Volunteer." Dedicated Andrew Crawford changed sheets, cleaned gurneys and did the scut work. Growing up, she learned to reach out to people in need. AIDS altered her feelings. She thought about contracting the disease in almost everything she did and when she reached out to help, it was with a gloved hand.

AIDS was never far from the minds of those who worked in the ER.

Regularly, Maines and her family discussed whether she should continue working where she did. The mother of three, she had only recently taken the hepatitis vaccine, and then only because of her kids. She still worried about the risks she took on the job. She knew that given "the kinds of people and issues we see every day, there's no way we can avoid accidents." But, she said, "ultimately, the patients are the reason we're there."

A distraught teenager with blond hair and bright red skin came in with her mother. Blowing on her arms, she complained she was on fire. Her mother said she was taking several medications, that she had been outside but only in the shade. The experienced nurse pointed out that if the redness came from anything other than the sun then it would have been all over her, including the backs of her arms. The nurse flipped over the teenager's arms. They were milky white.

Sometime after midnight a tough-looking teenager walked in, drawing instant attention. His upper lip looked like it has been mangled in a Cuisinart. Blood poured down his chin. Someone had gone after him with a golf club, he said. "A wood or an iron?" a nurse inquired. Immediately taken to a room, the teenager removed his shirt, revealing a beeper, the common form of communication for drug traffickers.

"What are you doing with that?" the nurse said.

"The girls call me," he responded. He had to have been in pain, but his only concern was relaying information to his buddies. The nurse refused. He didn't want deals consummated in the ER.

The difficult patient with the stab wound bounced around a gurney in the hallway. Whatever drug he had ingested was still operating. Periodically, he said that, no matter what, he was going to go to church on Sunday. Ro-chelle kept cropping up, too. "She's marked," he said. "Like God says, 'Man will destroy the world.' The flood. Forty-two days. Forty-two nights. The earthquake will take care of that . . . ."

Having no place to go, Mr. Comstock was informally invited to spend the night in the waiting room. When the police made their sweep, he knew the procedure—temporarily hiding in the parking lot.

The next night, when many of the same nurses were back at work, Mr. Comstock had a seizure in the parking lot and was returned to the hospital.

Last One In

AIDS patients didn't live in vacuum-packed communities. Disputes once limited to the General had begun to spill over into the public arena. The hospital's head of orthopedic surgery, Dr. Day, became the voice of doubt. On radio, TV and in print, she challenged the calm voices telling the public that sex, IV drugs and blood transfusions were the only means of contracting AIDS.

When Janet Pomeroy wanted to know about AIDS and swimming pools, she knew just whom she wanted to ask. But she didn't think so great a lady as Dr. Day would have the time to come to her Recreation Center for the Handicapped.

Thirty-five years earlier, Pomeroy had started the center, a unique facility, better known nationally and internationally than it was in San Francisco, its home city. The center was designed to provide recreational facilities for mentally and physically disabled people. A religious woman, Pomeroy began her work because, she said, "It was God's calling." From the time she was six, she knew she wanted to help people. In her teens, she'd searched until she found something she could give to others. She had begun on a small scale and, as California began emptying its mental hospitals, the center grew to accommodate the disabled suddenly sent to board-and-care homes or back to their families. By 1989, the remarkable center was helping eighteen hundred severely disabled people every week, offering arts and crafts, drama and sports, including swimming. Nevertheless, the center's good work was rarely acknowledged by city officials. In fact nobody paid much attention to it, hidden away in the cypress and pines in the southwest corner of the city, until the spring of 1989 when AIDS patients asked if they could swim in the center's pool.

The pool hovered at 92 to 95 degrees, warm enough for use by the elderly with arthritis or those with multiple sclerosis or cerebral palsy. The 115,000-gallon pool had built-in ramps for wheelchairs and gurneys and specially trained lifeguards to manipulate limbs for the handicapped.

Swimming supervisor Vince Huang received the request from two homes caring for AIDS patients. A tall, husky Asian with a wide face and freckles, Huang swam a mile in the Bay every morning before work. Active in liberal city politics, Huang would have invited the AIDS patients to swim at the center but he knew that the decision was not his to make. He referred the AIDS request to higher-ups.

"We didn't know enough about it," Pomeroy said. No one with a communicable disease had ever asked to swim. Pomeroy and the center were concerned about any potential "danger, particularly for children."

The center's letter responding to the request said it "recognizes the tragedy of AIDS," but that it didn't "know enough about how the AIDS virus might possibly be transmitted in a heated, therapeutic pool, especially to the young and elderly." Until it had more information, AIDS patients were not going to be permitted to swim. The letter continued: "The Center feels a need to consult with appropriate experts in the field."

With her blond pageboy, her oversize rose-rimmed sunglasses and lipstick to complement, Pomeroy resembled an aging movie star. And when she drifted through the grounds, she was greeted with respect by those who worked there and those who came to enjoy the facilities. Pleasantly eccentric, she shared her office with numerous cats. At home, she cared for more than a dozen others. Many, such as Jacob, Rachel and Rebecca, had biblical names.

A deeply religious woman, Pomeroy felt AIDS was a plague predicted in the Bible. When she lifted the Bible from the top drawer of her desk, it fell open to a page in Leviticus on "Penalties for Breaking the Law." In bright pink marker, she had bracketed the paragraph: "If a man lies with a male as he lies with a woman, both of them have committed an abomination; they shall surely be put to death. Their blood shall be upon them."

She seemed unaware that some staff members with whom she was close were gay and in one case had AIDS.

Pomeroy was pleased when Dr. Day agreed to speak both to the board of directors and to the parents of the handicapped. Day was unstintingly cooperative with the press or with any legitimate, sympathetic group. Of course, the more often she took to the public platform taking stands against the blood bank or against hospital policy, the greater was the cumulative anger toward her at the General.

Swimming supervisor Huang saw the issue spinning out of control. He dreaded what Day might say. He thought of her as something like Jim Jones of the Peoples Temple, a charismatic speaker adept at playing on people's fears. "It's like everything she says is the word of God. She's got that presence. She appears to have that type of power and persuasiveness."

At a well-attended meeting of parents whose children used the center, Day said she had "no information this disease can be transmitted through coughing or sneezing. However, I will tell you, nobody is looking at this. Nobody really wants to know if it can be transmitted."

She looked trim, fit. Her face was more than pretty. Yet it bore a hardness, brought on by the seriousness of her mission. She talked about her concern that the virus might be transmitted in sweat, from an infected person to a piece of exercise equipment and onto an uninfected person. Day regularly worked out at a gym.

But when she broached the issue with a medical epidemiologist at the CDC she was treated, she said, like she was a fool. She was told that AIDS could not be transmitted through sweat, even though, Day pointed out, the CDC had conducted no research to support its position.

From her argument with the CDC, Day moved onto the subject of pools.

"There are no recorded cases of anyone getting AIDS from a swimming pool," she continued. "Why? Because they haven't even looked at it. They have no information about it. They're doing it on the basis of no data. They assume that it you could get it through a swimming pool, everyone would have it. They assumed the same thing about sexual transmission and blood."

Day's words were confirming fears and weaving new ones. She acknowledged that chlorine probably kills the virus. But the problem, she said, was that "there will be areas of the swimming pool where you could have water that is in an area that chlorine doesn't get to." And the virus can live in water for a long time.

"Nobody's looked at the problem of body fluids being expressed in places close to another individual who does not have the virus. People urinate in a pool. The virus is in urine." And saliva, too, she said, can be expressed. "Patients with AIDS, particularly if they're far along in the disease, are incontinent." And, she added, "You may swallow some water."

The audience found the surgeon convincing, frightening.

She talked about what she called AIDS misinformation. "Anyone who speaks out is labeled a homophobic bigot. I am a doctor. I am only trying to save lives, gay or straight," she said.

"Nobody," she said, "wants to tell the truth. The government never wants to present to the American people a problem for which it has no solution. They do not have the guts to stand out and say, 'This is a war against a very bad disease and certain rights are going to have to be limited and we'll have to bite the bullet.' Nobody wants to do it because they won't get elected."

Her audience was with her.

City Hall, however, was not. Nor were the media. In a *San Francisco Examiner* article, Dr. George Rutherford, then chief of the San Francisco's AIDS office, countered Day: "There is no evidence that even remotely suggests this type of thing is possible."

Day spent about half an hour talking about swimming pools with one TV reporter. Aware that the reporter had recently had a child, Day went for the direct hit: "Why don't you take your new baby down there and swim in that pool with all those AIDS patients and someone gets a big glob of spit in the water and your baby swallows that. Is that all right with you?"

She told the reporter that AIDS patients had all the rights while people who don't have AIDS had none. "It would never happen that way in any other epidemic," Day said. But the quote that made it to the air was what Day said about "a big glob of spit."

If the pool controversy had been left to the parents, Day probably would have won. But there were other obstacles. Half the center's funding came from city coffers. And the five acres on which it sat were city owned, leased to the center for a dollar a year.

Representatives from the center were invited to meet with city human rights AIDS investigator Norm Nickens and city health officials. Dr. Alan Lifson, an MD with a master's in public health, one of the nation's experts on casual transmission of the disease, told the gathering that if the virus "was readily transmissible" through body fluids people who live in the same house with AIDS patients would be contracting the virus. In eleven household studies conducted so far, Lifson said, there had been no case of transmission through casual or household contact.

Near the end of Lifson's talk, Nickens asked about swimming and AIDS.

"Do you mean would I allow my three-year-old daughter to be in a pool with a person with AIDS?" Lifson asked. "Yes, I would. And have."

Daily, the tourniquet was tightening. Pomeroy and her board understood that if they made the wrong choice, they could lose their city funding.

The center received a letter from a member of the city's social service commission. The board member said that if discrimination against HIV-positive people did not end, he would try to cut off the $1.2 million the center received from the social service department each year. The letter writer added that "asking a fear-mongering crackpot like Day for counsel on AIDS is like turning to the Klan for advice on race relations."

By the end of May, the center's board had heard from the city's health department that HIV could not be transmitted in a swimming pool. The board voted unanimously to let people with AIDS use the pool.

"There was absolutely no choice," Pomeroy said. "The parents were unhappy. . . . [They] had worked so hard all these years. Everybody's worked so hard to get these facilities and then to have their place for their children to go, to have the city dictate what we can do and what we can't do, was a blow, particularly in terms of communicable disease. Everybody was saying there's absolutely no reason to be upset. So all that remains to be seen."

When the center's budget came up for review that year, the city ordered it to include mandatory classes on AIDS and homophobia.

The day of the first swim, swimming supervisor Huang anticipated trouble because he had paired AIDS patients with the elderly. Instead, he found the old people compassionate. It was, he said, as if they knew that the AIDS patients could be their children.

Still, harm had been done. Ten months after the incident, Huang looked out on an empty pool. During the time set aside for the once popular parent/child program for families in the neighborhood, no one showed. Whole cliques had quit coming. Other swimmers said they'd remain but they wouldn't put their faces in the water.

The absurdity of it impressed Huang. "What are people going to do? How do they know what's going on in their local pool? On vacation at the motel pool?"

Huang accepted the situation. New people were beginning to sign up. He didn't advertise the AIDS aspect. He thought about his daily swim in the Bay, amid garbage and sewage, and he reminded his swimmers, "You're here to swim in the water, not drink it."

To Pomeroy, Day remained her heroine: "She's a voice crying in the wilderness, a forerunner for the truth. She's not afraid to tell what she believes is true, and she's a doctor who knows what she's talking about."

Huang revised his views on the outspoken Day. After listening to her lecture, he no longer considered her a modern Jim Jones. He still felt she knew nothing about swimming pools: "We monitor the chlorine level in the pool very, very carefully." He continued to bring his two young daughters to swim. But other questions she raised impressed him. He wasn't sure he could teach AIDS 101 to the center staff any longer. He wasn't sure the AIDS experts knew what they were talking about anymore. Day was charismatic. She was just raising questions. Now, he was thinking Day was the medical profession's Ralph Nader.

The Way It's Supposed to Be

'll be in room ten for a while," the nurse told the desk. She shut the door, put some soft music on the radio and did what she felt was needed.

This is where men in their prime and those not yet in it came to heal temporarily, and this was where they came to die. For Nurse Sue Kiely, the deaths of young men had become as ordinary as the morning paper. She never knew what her patients did, who their mothers were or where they grew up. Here, they were stripped of life's accoutrements.

In earlier visits, the patient in Room 10 had insisted on meticulous cleanliness. After a night of spiking fever, he'd asked to wash off the sweat, shampoo his hair and use deodorant, even though he was receiving oxygen.

Now he was dying. But for his moans, he showed no expression. He'd lost consciousness two days before. He seemed to drift in and out; mostly out.

Having seen so many men in this condition, Nurse Kiely knew how frightened her patients were of pain and of death. Sometimes she rubbed their chests, in the place below the neck where her own chest tightened when she was frightened. Sometimes she just wiped a brow and listened. She thought she knew what might soothe this patient.

"I really think you would like to be clean right now," she said, approaching the hospital bed. He did not respond. Filling an umber bucket with warm water, she swirled in some Keri bath oil, purchased from the special AIDS fund to which the public frequently donated. With a washcloth in her right hand she grasped the patient's thumb, then his index finger, washing each finger as if he were her only patient. From the bony fingers, she moved to his whole hand and his wrist and then his forearm and elbow with the warm, silky water. As she went, she massaged his muscles and she spoke softly to him. When she finished one limb, she patted it dry, covered it and moved on to another. And when she completed a side, she stuffed pillows up against the bed rail, rolled the patient on his side and tucked in clean sheets.

Here at the AIDS inpatient unit known as 5A (the ward is on the fifth floor of the imposing main hospital building) Dr. Day's views were all but irrelevant. All of the patients were HIV positive and some of the staff was as well. Yet Kiely occasionally sympathized with a portion of what Day said and she recognized the risk of performing orthopedic surgery was greater than that of most other jobs at the hospital. She knew that as an AIDS nurse she, too, was taking some risk. She'd kept her fears under wraps until Jane Doe stuck herself. After that, Kiely could no longer ignore the risks.

She wasn't sure if she gave the bed bath for herself or for her patient. But doing it suited her and the unit. "You feel like a little kid when you're sick. You want your momma. You want someone to hold your head. That's how people feel when they're sick. I wouldn't imagine it's any different when you're sick with AIDS or when you're dying."

When the national media arrived in San Francisco to do AIDS stories, they came to the inpatient AIDS unit at the General to illustrate how it was supposed to be. Although it had only twenty private rooms and sometimes only enough nurses to serve sixteen of them, the AIDS unit came to be known as the ultimate example of AIDS care in the world. The floor plan, the nursing station and the rooms looked no different from any other ward at the hospital. But the place seemed airy, with butter-yellow and white walls; it appeared lighter. Large windows looked out over the hills of Twin Peaks and the city's Mission District.

The walls were decorated with patients' artwork. On one wall hung photographs of the nursing staff taken at the annual gay parade. And the unit's lounge had more amenities than others. Named the Elizabeth Taylor Lounge, after the star who has visited several times (insisting that there be no publicity), the lounge contained the piano she donated (on top of which sat a group photo of Taylor's wedding party), a ficus tree Taylor gave one year, other plants, a big-screen TV and a VCR.

Created in 1983 by Nurse Cliff Morrison, the AIDS unit was designed to give humane care to patients who'd been denied it elsewhere in the hospital. Ironically, Morrison had strongly opposed isolating AIDS patients. Appointed AIDS coordinator that same year, he felt one of his duties was to prevent the hospital from designating an AIDS ward. He figured he had enough influence to halt it and if he couldn't, as a gay man, he could galvanize the gay community to stop it. When the director of nursing broached the subject of opening a separate unit, Morrison balked but agreed to consider it.

Each day, as he visited AIDS patients throughout the hospital, he was appalled by the treatment they received. He found trays of dried and rotting food piled in corners, floors unwashed and unswept and wastebaskets brimming over. Feverish young men with nightsweats were unable to find nurses to change their soaked sheets or to bring them Tylenol. When bed linens were removed, they were thrown out. Frightened staff were posting signs on patients' doors—CONTAMINATED AREA. Many nurses wore gloves whenever they entered the room. One patient confided, "You don't know what it's like to only be touched by rubber."

The first member of his large, poor, Catholic family to finish high school and graduate from college, Morrison was raised by his mother, who worked in a hospital laundry. While openly gay, Morrison maintained close ties to his church.

One day, the deaf mother of a dying AIDS patient signed to one of the nurses that she wanted her son to have his last rites. The hospital priest arrived, observed the gowns, masks and gloves stationed outside the patient's room, and remarked, "He's got that gay disease, doesn't he?

"I'm sorry. I can't give him last rites," the priest said. "He brought it on himself."

The patient's nurse, Morrison and other Catholic nurses, who happened to be nearby, performed the last rites.

Perhaps more than any other, that incident led Morrison to believe that AIDS patients might need their own unit and their own staff.

He was not alone in his views. One of Volberding's patients with

Kaposi's sarcoma shared a room with one of the doctor's cancer patients, an older, black southerner, suffering from dementia. As if the KS patient weren't suffering enough, the older patient lectured him, saying he had sinned, that he had it coming, that he was suffering the curse of Job with pustules on the skin. The diatribe convinced Volberding that separating AIDS patients from the rest of the hospital population could be helpful.

When he discussed the plan with AIDS doctors in New York City that spring, they thought the concept was crazy. Nurses wouldn't want to work there. The house staff would try to avoid it. They warned him that he would be creating a unit for lepers.

Nurse Morrison, who teamed up with Volberding on the idea, went to the Shanti Project and to South of Market leather bars in search of patrons to support the idea. Morrison, like Volberding, had natural political instincts. Yet Morrison had no ambition—which worked to his advantage. He knew that a lot of men in the gay community opposed the idea of an AIDS ward, which sounded a lot like quarantine. He also knew that some of the hospital administrators, department heads and his peers were skeptical of it.

Creating an AIDS ward would violate nearly every nursing concept Morrison had been taught in school. He knew what he was doing was a risk. He also knew it was right. At thirty, he didn't really care who opposed the concept or what they thought. If it didn't work, he'd be unemployed and could always start over again.

It seemed surprising that a hospital, especially a teaching hospital, would give the authority to create such a controversial ward to a nurse. Morrison thought he understood why. Enough people agreed with him that something had to be done, but no one wanted to take the responsibility for it. They were willing to let him do it, he said, "mainly because they thought we wouldn't be able to accomplish anything."

Every day for three months, he rounded up the AIDS patients well enough to leave their beds, gingerly lowering them into wheelchairs, and pushed them to an empty ward on the fifth floor of the main hospital that would become the inpatient AIDS unit. Together, the dying men and the gay nurse designed the new facility.

When Morrison inquired, "What bothers you most about us?" the AIDS patients invariably responded, "Your arrogance. Your egos. You don't listen to us. You never approach us as humans."

Morrison determined that AIDS patients staying at the hospital would be taught about their disease and would make many of their own medical decisions, just as was being done in Ward 86, the AIDS outpatient unit. Everything in Morrison's unit was designed with the patients' needs, not that of the staff, in mind. Visitors were allowed to come any time. Patients were encouraged to bring things from home, to add warmth to institutional rooms. When early patients brought in crystal, wine, china, linen and an occasional candelabra, the AIDS unit earned an unfair reputation for snobbery. But what Morrison was doing helped turn the entire General around. Both destitute and well-off AIDS patients wanted to come to the county hospital.

One AIDS patient, unable to speak because he was on a ventilator, was visited by his mother, whom he hadn't had contact with in years. She stood in the doorway, arms outstretched with palms wrapped around either door molding and announced, "I'm in control here." To her son's lover she declared, "I don't want you in this room. That's how he got it. I don't want any of those homosexual doctors or nurses in this room. I am legally in charge of him. I will decide who comes into this room!"

After that, Morrison widened the definition of family. If he took his policy through committee, he suspected it would have been debated for months, maybe even years. He simply declared that henceforth AIDS patients would determine who their families were. Once the new family policy was publicized and praised, Morrison knew that the hospital administration wouldn't be likely to change it.

Another time, Morrison asked an AIDS patient, "Is there anything I can do for you?"

"What I want you to do you won't be able to do," the patient responded. "I want you to get in bed and hold me."

Morrison did.

The patient's regular nurse walked in, saw the AIDS nurse in bed, hugging the patient, and in shock, walked out. Various nurses complained about Morrison's unprofessional behavior. But his supervising nurse never objected. (Morrison had a protective shield with his powerful ally, San Francisco health director Dr. Mervyn Silverman. Silverman told the hospital to give Morrison anything he needed and he told Morrison that if he had any difficulty, just call. Morrison used the threat of calling Silverman sparingly. But many people went along with the nurse, knowing of his closely held clout.)

Many of the early patients were without family or a steady lover, and many died longing for human contact. When he formed the unit, Morrison worked against the nursing philosophy of distancing oneself from patients. He told his nurses to hold their patients' hands, to sit on their beds. He didn't expect them to lie down with everyone, but he wanted the nurses to know they had permission to do it and to hug a dying man if he needed to be hugged. He encouraged the nurses to cry. Tears, he said, were a sign of their strength and humanity.

Only nurses who volunteered for the unit were considered. It turned out that about half of the nurses were gay. Almost all, Morrison said with pride, were "troublemakers." Giving the nurses autonomy many of them hadn't sought, Morrison refused to name himself head nurse, preferring to be the coordinator. He insisted they work out their own schedules and settle problems among themselves. He served less as an authority figure and more as a role model. Because his AIDS unit was seen as such a risky concept, no one in the hospital was hovering over him. The unit was without a medical director for its first few years.

In many ways, AIDS is a nursing disease. Doctors couldn't cure AIDS patients, although they could control one opportunistic infection after another. In short order, the AIDS nurses became far more knowledgeable about the disease's many manifestations than were the medical students, interns and residents rotating through. An AIDS nurse might be seeing his seven-hundredth case of PCP while for a medical student, it might be his first.

San Franciscans regularly delivered gifts to the unit, which was known citywide as 5A. The San Francisco Tavern Guild, an organization of gay bar owners, contributed goody bags of toothbrush, toothpaste, body lotion, hairbrush, fleece-lined slippers and teddy bear to each AIDS patient. A refrigerator and VCRs were also donated. Smiling, camp Rita Rockett—cheerleader, chef, cancan and tap dancer and full-time altruist—cooked Sunday-night dinners, delivering them in her racy, mini black-and-white waitress uniform. Once a week "the cookie man" dropped by with shortbread cookies and pumpkin bread. "Some day," he told the nurses, "I may come down with AIDS. I want you to remember me." Just Desserts, a San Francisco–based baking company that uses only natural ingredients, brought cakes and other sweets daily. And Mrs. Fields sent over so many leftovers that it was rumored the bakers were purposely turning out dozens of extra chocolate-chip cookies every day.

In the early months there had been so much food that Morrison often invited other units to the daily buffet. As homophobic as some of the nurses and doctors were, as terrified of AIDS as they might have been, they nevertheless enjoyed the fruit salads, turkeys and cookies in the AIDS unit. Seizing on the opportunity, Morrison used the food to entertain and ensare people from whom he sought cooperation. In the beginning, nobody at the hospital was offering much more than skepticism. Morrison begged, bartered, coerced and outsmarted administrators. When he sought the help of Dr. Sande, director of medicine at the hospital, Morrison knew he could make Sande's life easier, and that if the inpatient AIDS unit worked, he could make Sande look good. "I let him take the credit," Morrison said. "It was a good bargain."

When Morrison wanted workers from the Shanti Project, where he was a volunteer, to help patients with their emotions or with physical problems, he called and suggested that Shanti propose it to the hospital administration. If the suggestion had come from him, Morrison felt certain it would have been vetoed. Following his suggestion, Shanti's leadership proposed placing its volunteers in the AIDS unit. When hospital officials consulted Morrison, he endorsed the Shanti proposal. Shanti workers became an integral part of AIDS care at the hospital. When housekeeping refused to mop up the unit, Morrison found money to offer the department two new job slots specifically for the AIDS inpatient unit. When dietary workers objected to bringing food to AIDS patients, Morrison, along with others, taught them what little was known about the disease, a course that had to be repeated over and over again as new employees were hired.

Morrison never sensed he was developing a model that would be replicated wherever good AIDS care is given. He wasn't even sure what the public reaction would be to the first AIDS unit anywhere until the media began coming by to do stories. The favorable pieces overcame any criticism of the unit. Morrison was impressed with how fast doubting administrators and politicians changed their minds, all making publicized pilgrimages to the AIDS unit to have their pictures taken there.

At times Morrison felt a nagging sense of guilt. He wondered how he could feel good when all around him there was so much sadness and death. Knowing he was making patients' lives better, seeing them live longer, he felt a sense of accomplishment.

The leper colony many feared constructing, never materialized. The unit came to be seen worldwide as the model of care. Morrison eventually was promoted to director of medical nursing, a position he thought he was given because he'd become too powerful in AIDS work. Nevertheless, he retained his position as AIDS coordinator. Weary of fighting for every little concession, assured the unit would survive, he left the General in 1986.

Over the years, doctors, nurses, politicians and celebrities have continued to flock to 5A. When she was still mayor, the tidy Dianne Feinstein was escorted to the new unit by Volberding. The two passed through the underground tunnels of the hospital, where they bumped into the hospital administrator and city health director Silverman. Just then, Feinstein spotted a pile of dust-covered vomit on the floor of the tunnel. She was told it would be cleaned up immediately. When she boarded the elevator, Feinstein winced at the graffiti on its walls. That, too, she was assured, would be taken care of pronto. Just as she reached the nursing station of the AIDS unit a wall behind her burst and a blast of steaming hot water shot across the floor like water from a hydrant on a hot summer's day. A pipe had broken. With sheets grabbed from the linen closet, janitors scurried around the mayor, soaking up the flood. Since then, celebrity visits have been smoother. Not long ago, Mother Teresa came at the request of former Mayor Agnos. She had showed up at his home one night—while he was out buying milk for his kids—to ask the mayor for an unused fire station for her soup kitchen. She took him to see the property and, in exchange, he took her to 5A to see the patients. After his advance people called to arrange for a minority patient to meet with him, Jesse Jackson came through the unit. Neither of the black patients on the unit had wanted to welcome him, but a Central American man, who'd not been out of bed in days, happily rose to greet Jackson.

The outpouring of love mingled with death. In a bathroom on 5A, someone had written DENIAL IS TERROR MANAGEMENT. And among the racks of information that line the front wall of the unit are brochures about funerals and cremations.

Like other nurses on 5A, Kiely grew used to sickness and death. It saturated her work and it was there when she went home to the Castro district, where delivery trucks dropped off tanks of oxygen and ambulances regularly raced to the neighborhood. Surviving meant that sometimes Kiely went numb. "You can't get a patient's IV line in," she said, "when you're sobbing all the time."

Struggling to maintain her idealism, sometimes, just sometimes, her fervor wavered. "I haven't cured anybody yet," she said, "and that's tough."

Sometimes she felt like a stand-up comic. She couldn't be on all the time. She couldn't perform to her fullest twelve hours of every working day without letup. On those days when she couldn't stand the suffering, instead of being Kiely, the loving nurse, she was just a good nurse.

In the early years, the unit experienced almost no turnover of its nursing staff. Back then, many patients came for therapy while complaining of boredom. Night nurses played checkers with their patients. But recent AIDS therapies allow patients to stay at home longer. Today, 5A patients are closer to death, and the nurses who care for them sometimes try to help them fall asleep when they're afraid they may not wake. Frequently nurses have to place bodies in zippered shrouds before having their morning coffee.

Before coming to 5A, one young nurse had worked in Calcutta for a couple of months, assisting Mother Teresa. She thought she understood death. "But I really didn't understand the scope of the AIDS virus: how young they were, how much they hurt, how little can be done for them, how short their life spans were, how quickly it came on, how devastating it was."

She sometimes found it analogous to the shock of war, and she thought most people didn't experience the bundle of emotions she felt until they reached old age.

The hardest part was that "people are suffering and they want to live," she said. "They're full of life and they're dying." Helplessly she watched as an artist lost his sight, a musician his hearing or someone who was independent his ability to walk. She might work hard to help a patient walk out of 5A, only to see him return six months later to die.

Like the other nurses on the unit, she tried to allow her patients to die with dignity, which meant without a lot of futile medical intervention. She just wanted to help the patient reconcile his life and die in peace. She did it by listening, and sometimes by calling in a Shanti worker to help, and sometimes just by holding on. In her melodic voice she said, "All a person needs sometimes is a touch or a word or a look. It's probably what they were looking for their whole lives anyway."

AIDS hadn't crushed her philosophy. She still believed that for every problem there must be a solution. She failed to understand why curing AIDS should take so long. She understood the medical reasons. Still, she said, "I want these people to get cured. I don't care why they're dying. I just don't want them to die anymore."

Although nursing at 5A is considered the pinnacle of the profession, some nurses have begun to leave. Some have gone back to school, had babies or decided to work elsewhere. A few gay nurses have become ill with AIDS. The pressure, already there, has increased, as nurses are caring for fewer middle-class gay patients.

"People are on this ward to take care of AIDS patients," said one of the unit's supernurses. "But really, we're here to take care of gay AIDS patients." (Many other 5A nurses didn't feel the way she did. Nurse Alise Martinez, for example, came not because the patients were gay but because theirs was a new disease and because she wanted to care for people others were afraid to care for.) She was drawn to 5A because she knew she was needed there. Patients appreciated her.

As AIDS spread into the drug-using population, the 5A nurses found themselves caring for patients whose last home was a sidewalk. Some were angry at everyone, including the selfless nurses. When she described the two groups, generalizing to make her point, the supernurse thought about the appreciative, well-informed gay patients and the extreme IV drug-using ones who sometimes told her, "Fuck you. I'm not going to do anything you tell me to do, bitch." Some of them have tried to stuff their hands down narrow-necked Sharps boxes to retrieve used needles. Others have demanded more pain medications. Nurses were having to call hospital security more often.

Once, when the supernurse went to care for a drug addict AIDS patient, his sixteen-year-old-daughter confronted her: " 'What the fuck are you doing for my father?' " Times like that, she had to remind herself why she was there. She told the daughter she understood how frightening it must be for her to see her father so ill.

Despite the loving dispositions of the AIDS nurses, with some of the IV drug-using population, they found they could no longer be unconditionally caring. Having grown used to patients they could have fun with and whose psychic pain they could lessen, they sometimes felt uncomfortable with some of the new population. They wanted it to be the way it had been.

As chronic rescuers, they felt guilty disliking some of these difficult patients. Many of the IV drug-using patients were good patients. But when the cantankerous, sometimes treacherous ones were hostile or threatening, the nurses wanted to retreat. "We do what we need to do," a nurse said, "but it isn't sitting on the bed holding a hand."

Being a nurse at 5A was Tony Lobb's way of being there for his community. He'd grown up in rural Kentucky with an inborn sense of patriotism. If there'd been a war, Tony would have enlisted. But when he got to 5A, "it wasn't my community or what I perceived to be my community." Sometimes the IV drug-using population resented Lobb's Truman Capote-esque mannerisms, his calling patients "honey." While most patients assigned to 5A and their friends were pleased to get a room there, some drug-using patients didn't want to be associated with the unit. One screaming man, clutching his fake Luis Vuitton purse as he was being wheeled on a gurney into 5A at 1:30 A.M., pulled himself up long enough to holler in his falsetto voice: "I be's a bisexual! I be's a bisexual!"—presumably, a cut above a gay.

Nurse Lobb longed for what he thought of as the stereotypical AIDS patient: sweet, handsome, knowledgeable and appreciative. Sometimes even when he did care for such patients, he found the work upsetting. Too often, they were tangled in tubes with no hope of living very long and believed they were at the hospital for the big fix. In time, Lobb came to feel he was presiding over death.

Having been tested for HIV, he knew he was negative. He felt survivor's guilt and he felt as if he were being left behind. That he could do so little gnawed at him. "What do I say to these people when they're reaching out, wanting hope and wanting a cure? And I know I can get them through part of it. I can't do anything in the long run. It's so hard. It's so hard to go in every day."

In some ways, working at 5A was anathema to nursing. "The things I do as a nurse are to keep people alive," he said.

For Nurse Kiely, 5A was nursing the way it was supposed to be. But she knew that if she weren't watchful, her profession could bleed her dry. More and more, she found herself working her three-day, twelve-hour shifts, going home, pouring herself into a hot bath and healing for four days so she could return to work. Days off she had to close up the psychic wounds of patients who'd affected her. At a café, she'd sip coffee but not talk to other people. The longer Kiely worked at 5A, the weaker were her defenses.

She used to call her patients her "babies." Men who might have been friends outside the hospital became her friends in the ward. Their deaths hurt her more than those of the others. Over two months, a cluster of her favorite patients died, leaving Kiely feeling like a raw nerve rubbed up against a wire brush.

Hating funerals, Kiely rarely went to one. But one Sunday, when she tagged along with a friend visiting a dying man with AIDS, the sick man died. As were his wishes, his friends gathered around his body to reminisce. She hadn't allowed herself to mourn until then. She cried for the friend of a friend who'd just died. And she cried for all the people she'd never shed tears for. "All these people who died with me."

Rolling Thunder

They came at him like rolling thunder—accusing, denigrating, demanding that he account for his science. This should have been Dr. Michael McGrath's finest hour. The discoverer of Q had completed a speech to AIDS activists, giving them the most optimistic news in a long time. Then it happened. As he disappeared behind the stage, a handful of ACT UP (the AIDS Coalition to Unleash Power) members pressed in around him.

"Why didn't you tell people in 1987 about this incredible drug?"

"Why did you wait until your findings were published in April of 1989?"

"You knew about this for two years and the same drug was available in China! A lot of people died during those two years."

"Why were there delays?"

"What's the difference between your drug and Chinese Q?"

"My lover died and he could have had this drug!"

Activists referred to a sheet of paper on which were written dates:

when the patent for GLQ223 was filed, when it was issued, when the *Proceedings of the National Science Academy* published McGrath's findings on Q.

He explained that there were no delays. That he did not know the purity of the drug from China. That he'd never been able to get more than a small quantity of it from Dr. Yeung, the Hong Kong scientist who had brought it to him in the fall of 1986. That he and his collaborators at Genelabs had spent a year and a half conducting animal toxicology studies, as required by the Food and Drug Administration.

The activists accused McGrath of pursuing profits over lives. By maintaining an early silence he'd adhered to the scientific etiquette followed by all reputable academics. Refusing to discuss one's research prior to publication is part of the brotherly code of science that weeds out inaccuracies through an elaborate review-and-validation process.

The quick, affable scientist/physician had agreed to speak to the annual HIV Treatment Awareness meeting in San Francisco. Organized by Project Inform, the AIDS advocacy and information organization, the meeting brought McGrath together with angered AIDS advocates from around the nation.

Only a few weeks before, news had broken about the most promising drug since the advent of the epidemic. While maintaining their skepticism, AIDS patients began to think the impossible: that there might be a cure. In 5A, Nurse Sue Kiely's excitement was salted with doubt. Was it really working? Or was it another exaggerated prospect?

At the community speech held in San Francisco's large civic auditorium, McGrath talked about what Q could do in a petri dish—kill infected cells while leaving healthy ones alone. But he warned that what happened in vitro did not always occur in vivo (in the living body). And he advised his audience not to risk infusing themselves with the root of cucumber. Rumors were circulating that a few AIDS patients had gotten hold of a Chinese root and ingested it, nearly killing themselves. But for the most part, McGrath's message was upbeat.

One of the AIDS activists, Terry Beswick, had already read about McGrath's experiments. What impressed Beswick now was the fact that the young scientist, with no background in politics, had accepted the invitation to speak. That alone set him apart from other doctors at San Francisco General who shelled up like turtles in a sandstorm, refusing to talk about Q.

But in the new world of AIDS, ACT UP demonstrators often wore black T-shirts with pink triangles reading: SILENCE-DEATH.

As with the other activists, first-year medical student Michelle Roland, one of the people haranguing McGrath, thought scientific silence was criminal when thousands were dying. "It's the people's right to choose," she told McGrath. "If there's information, put it out there."

"Listen, I'm a doctor," McGrath told the group. "I take care of patients and they're dying. Q just wasn't ready." Most scientists work in societal isolation, in labs distant from the people they're trying to help. By working at the General, McGrath had no chance to distance himself from the people he was trying to help. He didn't tell the activists confronting him that sometimes in the course of his experiments he had been haunted by the vials of Q on his lab counter and by the trail of wasted men dragging themselves to Ward 86, the outpatient AIDS unit.

"The worst thing you can do to a drug is give it a bad rap," he said to the angered activists, just before he was to gain firsthand knowledge. "If information about Q had leaked out while animal toxicology studies were being conducted, if AIDS patients had experimented on themselves and died, Q would have been finished before it started. The gay community would label it 'gasoline' and it would never be heard from again. People would say 'It's a poison,' and the fact is, it is poison. They would say 'It kills people.' And it could. And that would be the death of Q," McGrath told them. "There's a reason for doing it quietly."

The incident might have grown nastier but for the spreading word that McGrath was sympathetic to the activists' cause. ACT UP members had been considering other actions against the University of California Medical School at San Francisco for keeping the Q data secret for two years. But they took it easy on McGrath. "We sensed that McGrath was a good guy," Roland said. "We didn't want to trash him."

The day he'd made his findings public, McGrath had received a phone call from Martin Delaney, the pied piper of Project Inform. Delaney quizzed the scientist about his findings. The call from the forty-three-year-old Delaney, a former Jesuit seminarian, marked the beginning of a highly controversial relationship between the university scientist and the radical AIDS activist.

Later that day, McGrath spoke to a meeting of AIDS activists organized by Donald Abrams, one of the top AIDS doctors at the General. Delaney appeared at the meeting, handing out his just-written fact sheet on Q. Incredible, McGrath thought. He can put words to paper faster than anyone I've ever heard of. He's accurate. And he can parrot everything that is said.

As news of Q spread, activists knew where to find McGrath. Many adhered to a conspiracy theory. Others were even harsher.

"I am a mass murderer," McGrath told his staff on returning from one difficult newspaper interview. As it often did, McGrath's irony unnerved researcher Isabelle Gaston and the others in his lab. There were times when Gaston had been impatient with the pace of research—her own as well as others'. Friends were dying. But she couldn't imagine anyone attacking McGrath.

"What?" McGrath went on. "You didn't know you were working for a killer?"

A journalist from a gay newspaper had waited until he had finished interviewing McGrath before springing his own accusation. He asked McGrath what it felt like to withhold news about a drug that could have saved thousands of lives.

These were difficult times for the ebullient researcher. It was only the start. Like Styrofoam on a wave, McGrath and Q were about to be buffeted by media winds and gay sentiment. Unlike some of the doctors at the General who had been active in antiwar politics in the sixties and who remained political, McGrath, at thirty-six, had never weathered political storms. Having discovered Q and conducted early experiments, suddenly he found himself in one of the angriest political thickets. He was baffled.

The explanation was inherent in the drug. Q offered greater promise than any other drug. It was cheap, available (from China) and organic.

The news accounts began appearing in early 1989 with the publication of the patent for Q. A little blurb ran in the Saturday Patent column of the *New York Times*, just above one for Ampligen, a drug thought to be useful in the fight against AIDS until it was tested in humans, and another for aluminum mulch that reflects sunlight, enabling plants to grow better.

Local reporters wanted to know if McGrath had suppressed information. He said nothing. For three or four weeks he observed a news embargo while waiting for the article about Q to be published in the *Proceedings of the National Academy of Science*.

On April 13, the day the Q article was published, the embargo was lifted. Telephone lines to the General's public-relations office jammed.

Calls were coming in from England, Australia and all over the United States. McGrath's lab became what he called "blitz city." Cameras and lights were squished into narrow walkways. Telephones rang. Researchers found it difficult to maneuver around the lab. But McGrath did his best to accommodate. Later, he was chagrined to find photographs of himself in a lab coat holding up test tubes without wearing gloves.

The Italian equivalent of *Nightline* flew in from Milan on a Saturday. McGrath wanted to be home but the crew threatened suicide if he didn't show. He obliged, apologizing for his laryngitis. The Italian director of the show said McGrath's voice didn't matter. "We're going to dub you in Italian." The Italian crew carried a bag of three kinds of cucumbers. "Which one is it?" they asked. "Could you hold it up?"

"It's not the cucumber," McGrath said.

"It's not?" Italians with AIDS, the crew told him, were making cucumber extract and eating and injecting it.

It was not the cucumber McGrath was studying but the purified protein from the root of the Chinese cucumber. So on that Saturday, he did a little Italian public education.

One San Francisco TV reporter conducted an interview with him, closing the piece outside a Chinatown market. The reporter held up a bitter melon, presumably the type from which came Q's cousin, momorcharin, an extract derived from the seeds of bitter melon, and cautioned viewers not to try to purify the compound themselves. The scene appalled the scientist: "There she was, holding it up for everybody to see."

McGrath intuitively knew what the Reagan and later Bush White House understood, that what people see carries greater weight than what they might hear. He worried that desperate people might descend on Chinatown, buy something resembling Q and inject themselves. "If you go to Chinatown and get hold of these materials or their extracts, they won't work and could cause a tremendous amount of harm," he advised reporters.

By comparison, the *New York Times*'s first article on Q (after the announcement of the patent) was conservative, appearing on page 6 of the science section, headlined EARLY TESTS PROMISING FOR A NEW AIDS DRUG. The piece included drawings of the Chinese plants and roots and a picture of a gloved McGrath with test tube.

The *Village Voice* led with a cover article headline that read Q: CAN

THIS DRUG STOP AIDS? Newspaper columnists called it a possible cure. The gay press—with the exception of the accusatory pieces—fell into an optimistic frenzy. Despite his own ingrained optimism, McGrath was more cautious. At the time these articles were appearing, he was saying that if human trials went well he imagined Q being used for what an oncologist would call induction therapy, to kill off most of the HIV-infected cells. Because Q is a protein and a toxin, it could not be given for long periods of time. McGrath imagined additional therapy to include a nontoxic medicine to block reinfection of cells. "Even if you are getting rid of ninety-nine-point-nine percent of the HIV-infected cells, you are going to have a few left over. There will probably always be the need for treatment with something."

Cautiously, researchers at the General made plans to test GLQ223 on willing patients.

The Right Thing to Do

At 3 A.M. on a warm, spring Sunday, Dr. Bill Schecter tugged on his black ranch boots, lowered his welder's mask, wrapped a waterproof apron around himself and double gloved. In the operating room, the patient's body lay on the cold steel table, covered in blood-soaked hospital linen. Blood puddled on the linoleum and seeped outward like ink across a blotter. It sprayed out, splashing onto a resident's elbow, leaving a large pancake-size stain. It smudged a nurse's wrist. Gloves and gowns of the residents, nurses and Schecter were marbled dark red.

Here in the operating room, the blurred debate over a physician's responsibility came into focus. Everyone who scrubbed for an operation was at risk. Every eight years, someone in the General's operating room was expected to contract the AIDS virus on the job, according to a study conducted by Dr. Gerberding, head of the hospital's massive health-care workers study. A lot of busy surgeons suspected the figures would go much higher.

No one knew the name of the patient on the operating-room table, let alone his HIV status. In trauma surgery, there was no time to find out. A few minutes after the bars closed on Saturday night he'd been stabbed in the neck and had lost so much blood that by the time the white-and-orange ambulance backed into the emergency-room entrance the patient was clinically dead. Blood cascaded out the back of the ambulance as paramedics kicked open the door. They grabbed the gurney and shot down the hospital corridor. Patients, nurses and cops shoved themselves up against the wall as the gurney, dripping blood, raced by.

In the trauma room, a short nurse leaped onto a stool and rhythmically pressed the patient's heart. With a special scalpel, a resident—so rushed he hadn't time to put on his surgical gown—sliced through the patient's skin and pericardium, the lining of the heart. He pulled the heart out and kneaded it like dough. His gloved hands were bloodied.

If given the choice, even the liberal attending surgeon, a role model for many residents, would not want to operate on someone who could give him a fatal disease. Like many of his colleagues, he's been stuck by a needle full of HIV-positive blood. And like many of them, he has not been tested because, he said, "That's not something I want to know."

"I'm not crazy," Schecter told medical students. He didn't want to take unnecessary risks. But that was his job. "When you're in the middle of a firefight, you've got to do what you have to do."

A machine pumped blood into the patient as fast as his body could absorb it. Blood had drained from his vessels. His organs were dying. The brain could only survive for four minutes without the flow of oxygen-saturated blood.

As the surgeons probed for the cause of the massive hemorrhage, Schecter reached into the open chest and cradled the patient's heart in his hands. Operating-room lights bounced off the muscle as he squeezed it repeatedly, trying to force blood out. With his hands he tried to do what the normal heart does by beating: push blood into the coronary arteries.

Schecter was the philosophical antithesis of Dr. Day. When reporters needed someone to counter her claims, they sought Bill Schecter. One of his peers praised him by saying he had the soul of a nurse. To many, he'd become the conscience of the county hospital.

AIDS made surgeons more careful. When doctors and nurses in the operating room passed instruments, they placed them in kidney basins or on stands to lessen the chance of a stick. When they could, many doctors preferred to shoot surgical staples into skin rather than suture an incision and risk a prick. And when an operation such as the one they were performing required cauterization, the smoke could be removed by a smoke evacuator. No one knew for sure whether HIV could be transmitted by smoke. Schecter didn't want to be the index case that others wrote about.

He balanced the risk with his sense of responsibility. Reaching as he often did for a military metaphor, Schecter likened surgeons to troops in the Special Forces. Surgeons hold an elite position in society. They have special knowledge and they violate society's taboos. They cut people open. They put their hands inside them. People tell them things they wouldn't confide to anyone else. Men and women take off their clothes and allow surgeons to examine them. By entering a profession with prestige and with secret knowledge, Schecter told doctors-to-be they were giving up a risk-free environment.

When debates raged in hospital committee meetings, Schecter often quoted from the Old Testament and from the writings of early physicians. Although not religious in the traditional sense, it was in the history of the Jewish people that he found answers.

While the more powerful Day, head of orthopedic surgery, was talking about providing alternatives to surgery and testing patients for the virus, Schecter reduced the argument to what he saw as its essence. If it benefited the patient, he said, he'd perform surgery. He turned to Leviticus, which said, "Neither shalt thou stand idly by the blood of thy neighbor."

While Day was on sabbatical in 1989–90, giving speeches about physicians' rights, Schecter and pediatric surgical specialist Dr. Michael Harrison operated on a five-year-old Russian boy with the AIDS virus. Born with a perforated anus, at the age of two the boy had undergone unsuccessful corrective surgery, during which he had been transfused with AIDS-contaminated blood. After that no one in the then Soviet Union was eager to operate on him again. Isolated and ill, the child's stool was leaking from his body. He was chronically infected. Brought to the attention of the Center for Attitudinal Healing, an organization based in Marin County, the boy was flown from his home in Smolensk to San Francisco. When asked to help the child, Schecter replied, "Sure. I'll operate on anybody."

On Presidents' Day, a day off for the physicians, Schecter and colleagues operated for eight and a half hours. They agreed to do the operation free of charge. (The city of San Francisco paid for the boy's hospital stay.) At considerable risk to themselves, the surgeons disconnected the rectum from the urethra. The boy spent less than two weeks in the hospital before being moved to a Catholic Charities facility with his mother. He was no longer incontinent or infected from his stool. He became healthier and was able to lead a more normal life and eventually return home.

Schecter and his colleagues operated "on the kid who was HIV positive," because, he said, "it was the right thing to do."

When he was a college student, Schecter had imagined himself a statesman or a military leader, but the Vietnam War altered his perspective. He had been influenced by an Israeli short story by Aaron Meged he read in Hebrew (Schecter also is fluent in Spanish and French). In the story, an army officer, who'd fought in Jerusalem in the war of independence, had thought he'd do something significant with his life. After the war, he married, had two children and took a Tel Aviv office job. Returning to Jerusalem, he visited his old girlfriend and wandered the Judean hills. After three days, he boarded the bus back to Tel Aviv. His wife said nothing. He said nothing. The next morning, he rode the bus back to the office.

Schecter determined that his life was never going to be as ordinary as that of the Israeli army officer. Early in his academic career, Schecter had been branded a maverick. Right after their internship, he and his wife, Gisela, who now heads the busy TB clinic at the General, had taken a nine-hundred-mile canoe trip to the Arctic Ocean. From 1981 to 1983, Schecter was chief of surgery at the LBJ Tropical Medical Center in Pago Pago, American Samoa. There he was able to recreate the surgical training of some of his teachers who had grown up doing everything, before specialization limited surgeons to narrower fields of expertise. Methodically, Schecter had chosen Pago Pago because it was farther from any medical center than was any other place in the world. It took six hours by jet to reach the nearest hospital. When patients showed up, it would have been unethical for Schecter not to care for them. He did neurosurgery and orthopedic surgery. He did cleft palate surgery and many craniotomies (opening the skull to operate on the brain). He did reconstructive hand surgery for leprosy patients.

In the upward-mobility track at UC Medical School doctors focused on one area and tried to advance knowledge in it. Schecter continued to steer in the opposite direction. So while others were jockeying for better positions, he and his physician wife took off for a South African hospital with an integrated faculty and staff that served black, Indian and colored patients. The hospital was a referral center for twenty million people. On the wards, desperately ill patients were more concerned with getting well than with politics.

Even when he came back to California, Schecter never lived the ordinary life. Each morning, he left home in Half Moon Bay, a sleepy coastal town, and swam in the icy bay before driving to work. On Mondays, when patients came to the outpatient clinic, he zigzagged from exam room to exam room and from drama to drama. One patient, who had seen the sign of Satan in his hand, had sliced it off; Schecter had reattached it. Another had come through the emergency room in shock with a hole in his colon and stool floating around in his abdomen. Schecter operated on him and would operate again. The surgeon was proud of the fact that at the General "We don't do a 'wallet biopsy' before deciding who to treat." He examined a softspoken woman whose finger was infected—the result of a human bite, a common injury. Schecter examined lumps in the breasts of a scared Chinese mother who wanted to go home for her son's birthday; an old Arabic woman with a face creased like a raisin; a stressed-out black teenager who mistook her own rib for a lump. And he cajoled a pleasantly nutty patient with a loud, cheery voice who came by nearly every Monday just to chat with the friend she calls "Dr. Schecker"!

In the early '80s, AIDS was something that didn't concern surgeons. Policy was made by infectious-disease doctors and oncologists and by administrators with social and political agendas. Surgeons were told they needn't worry . . . just be careful. Schecter headed the General's operating-room committee that declared in early 1987 that blood was to be considered a toxin. Stricter protective procedures were advised. After Jane Doe seroconverted, Schecter began the tedious task of working with the hospital, the city and the university to increase compensation for the next nurse or doctor who contracted the AIDS virus on the job. The present amount, Schecter said, wouldn't keep his kid in comics.

Initially the Centers for Disease Control and local researchers characterized physicians' risk of contracting the disease as "low." As a very busy surgeon who sometimes stuck himself, Schecter wouldn't use the word *low*. "We may not be epidemiologists," he said, "but we're also not schmucks." Both Schecter and Day were irritated by the CDC's cavalier attitude. Day's fury, Schecter felt, stemmed from the fact that she expected the very best in people. With five-thousand years of Jewish history to rely on, he had come to expect the very worst.

Being Jewish had served him well. A friend of his once said that Jews were not genetically designed to work for salaries. And while the surgeon was salaried and working for an academic hierarchy, he was in it but not of it. He remained the outsider. His identity came not from his status at the university but from his culture and family.

For new doctors looking for guidance or searching for role models other than Lorraine Day, Schecter, an associate clinical professor of surgery at UCSF, gave them answers. While Day's manner was forceful, sometimes angry, his was calm. Day dealt with immediate risks and immediate fears; Schecter's views were more historical.

When Schecter was asked to speak to medical students or surgeons about practicing surgery in a hospital clogged with AIDS patients, he told them there was plenty of precedent for walking away from an epidemic. At the time of the Black Plague, the Greek physician and writer, Galen, fled Rome rather than treat patients. Most of the physicians in Venice fled as well. Of those who stayed, many locked themselves in their homes.

At a gathering of Jewish medical students, he read a passage by Guy de Chauliac, one of Pope Clement VII's surgeons, which he thought they might find meaningful: "They dared not visit the sick, for fear of becoming infected. And when they did visit, they did nothing, and earned nothing, for all the sick died. . . . To survive, there was nothing better than to flee the region before becoming infected. . . . And I, to avoid infamy, did not dare remove myself, but with continuous fear preserved myself as best I could. . . ."

Then Schecter gave them examples of people who had risked their lives to care for the sick. He quoted from the memoirs of apothecary William Boghurst on the plague in 1666: "Every man that undertakes to bee of a profession or takes upon him any office must take all parts of it, the good and the evill, the pleasure and the pain, the profit and the inconvenience altogether, and not pick and chuse; for ministers must preach, Captains must fight, Physitians attend upon the Sick . . ."

In his talk to medical students, Schecter explained the muddied message of the American Medical Association. In 1846, the newly formed organization stated in its code of medical ethics that it was the physician's duty to face the danger of pestilence and to continue his labors (and to continue) suffering even at the jeopardy to their own lives. But in 1957, the code was shortened and that segment was deleted. The 1980 version of the AMA's principle of medical ethics, Schecter felt, read "more like a commercial contract rather than a standard for the highest moral behavior of a profession."

Schecter tried to convince his audience to treat HIV-positive patients because it was the right thing to do. "Failure to treat these patients," he told them, "is a serious moral lapse based upon the professional requirements of virtue, duty and compassion for our fellow man."

At the same time, he encouraged students to take precautions. When he gave a talk in Stockholm on infection-control precautions to an international conference on blood-borne infections, he was asked by a member of the audience how much the precautions cost and if they were really worth it.

If he were an administrator in Zaire, who had "a limited amount of money and I was trying to decide whether to buy more gloves for doctors in the hospital or spend my money on water-pollution control and immunization programs for the population, I might make one decision. If I happened to be the doctor working on the ward, I'd make another decision. I said basically, what you're asking is 'How much is the life of a single health-care worker worth?' And my response to that is that if it happens to be my life, it's worth an infinite amount of money!" After this speech, he would laugh.

A student wanted to know if his morality waned after working a solid forty-eight hours. He told the students about his experiences in South Africa where one day, after intratribal strife, seventy-two patients were admitted to the surgery service and he did fifteen laparotomies (abdominal operations) in twenty-four hours. He didn't answer the question directly but instead told the student what he tells his residents. When he dies, they can put this on his tombstone: HE DID THE BEST HE COULD—UNDER THE CIRCUMSTANCES.

Foxhole

People at the General felt Dr. Day's unspoken message was to abandon AIDS patients, although she always denied it. In 1989, she received a syringe and a needle with AIDS-contaminated blood in it through the mail. The anonymous critic wrote that he hoped she would stick herself with it. Often the attack was more sophisticated. Before Day spoke at a conference in Australia, a committee of Australian federal and state officials issued a white paper refuting each point it expected her to make.

Meanwhile the battle at the hospital raged on, although the debate centered around a physician's right to test patients rather than the more critical one of a physician's responsibility to treat patients.

By the spring of 1989, Day's opponents had appealed to the university hierarchy, without success. Worried that she might not treat all HIV-infected patients, the physicians wrote a new bylaw for the General. Pegged "the Lorraine Day clause," it stated that the hospital must provide all needed medically appropriate care for all patients regardless of race, sex, creed or current medical condition. With its enactment, the bylaw marked the start of what could have become adversarial proceedings against Day.

She had been fighting the hospital establishment for two years, and the skirmishes had turned her into a different person. She felt like a soldier in a foxhole. "You cannot be constantly ground down by your peers," she said, "and not have it affect you."

If she continued to perform orthopedic surgery at the General, where one out of four surgery patients was HIV positive, she believed she was likely to contract the virus. In a June 23, 1988, *New England Journal of Medicine* article, Day's personal risk of seroconversion was estimated to be 49 percent in five years. The findings were based on her own estimates that she received forty needle-sticks per year and that a third of the sticks contained blood from HIV-positive patients. Her critics, well versed in health-care workers' safety, contended that forty sticks a year was an extraordinarily high estimate.

The real issue, some of her colleagues felt, wasn't so much a doctor's right to test for AIDS as it was her fear of the disease. For as long as she was willing to operate on trauma patients (she always was) who are raced into the operating room without time to test for AIDS, she was going to be at risk. Chief of staff Dr. John Luce, with whom she often sparred, felt she either was going to have to work at the General "and stop worrying about all this HIV testing or [she's] got to leave."

She had pretty much reached the same conclusion. Nevertheless, while on sabbatical in 1989, Day returned to the General. While, as she put it, "still trying to get common sense into these knuckleheads," she took her case to a much larger arena. Her vehicle would be an appearance on *60 Minutes*.

The TV crew lunched on rolls and coldcuts brought in by Day's devoted gay secretary. A second-generation vegetarian, Day was not partaking. While they sipped cans of soda and schmoozed in cubicles outside her office, Day rushed away to console the patient who the CBS producer, reporter, cameraman and soundman had come to film: a patient requiring a bloody operation and thought possibly to be HIV positive. Not just any surgical patient would do. The *60 Minutes* crew had flown in from New York on this prearranged day for the prearranged operation they requested to observe. They wanted to document the risks that Day felt she and the residents and nurses were taking. And they wanted to show her operating in her space suit.

Minutes before the operation, the patient was crying. She wanted to go home. The cause of her anxiety was the IV needle. She'd come to the hospital in constant pain. She walked only with difficulty. A car accident and subsequent surgery had left her with fractures in the bone between her ankle and knee that had never properly healed (bilateral nonunion fractures of the tibias). Treated at another hospital with plates and screws in her legs, she came to the General in search of greater mobility and less pain. Day planned to replace the rods, hoping to stimulate the bone to heal properly. It was a sufficiently bloody operation for the 60 *Minutes* crew to get what Day called "a good flavor." But at this moment, the patient, an alcoholic and possibly a heroin addict, just wanted to forget about the whole thing. Away from the media, Day calmed her, promising to give her anesthesia before putting in the IV. Returning to the TV crew stationed outside her office, Day announced, "The lady was putting us up against the wall."

The patient's HIV test had come back negative, but with that window of chance, between the time one acquires the virus and one tests positive, the risk to the operating room staff remained. (The June 1, 1989, *New England Journal of Medicine* documented cases in which men had been exposed to the virus but had not tested positive for as long as three years afterward.) She might carry the virus, so Day and her residents would have to wear their space suits.

This was Jeff Fager's first season as a producer on 60 *Minutes*—he'd moved over from *West 57th Street*—and this was his best piece to date. Frank and eloquent, Day was saying what a lot of physicians nationwide were thinking and fearing. The son of a brain surgeon, Fager appreciated the issue's importance—Day's directness astonished and pleased him.

Fager never had to wrestle with the hospital's PR staff the way other producers and reporters seeking access to the General had to. Having tangled with Day before, the PR women left the 60 *Minutes* crew alone.

Not only were reporters coming to her at the General, but in recent months Day had become the lead speaker on the surgical circuit worldwide. While her talks were full of statistics, they were heavy on the drama. She often targeted the bureaucrats: "It's easy to tell someone what risks to take in life when they're sitting there smug in their offices, pushing paper," she would tell them. "They're up in their penthouse like generals in world war, deciding who they're going to sacrifice on the front line. When the war is over, we'll all be dead and they'll be riding in the parade."

In her conversation with 60 Minutes reporter Steve Kroft, Day spoke about her concerns. "Our risk is one in two hundred per needle-stick of AIDS blood," she said, using the established figures. (More recently, the CDC has estimated the risk to be one in three hundred and thirty-three per needle-stick.) She went on, "If you come to work every day and flicked the light switch on in your office and only one out of two hundred times you were electrocuted, would you consider that low risk?" The analogy seemed shaky, since people walk in a room and flick on the lights more often than surgeons operate or cut themselves. Nevertheless, it made for effective TV.

Day compared the risk of performing surgery with that of having anal sex. Interviewed by 60 Minutes, the federal Centers for Disease Control's Jim Curran agreed that the risk of contracting the AIDS virus from one needle-stick (with AIDS blood) was about equal to the risk of engaging in one act of anal sex. Curran admitted that the CDC's figures for the number of health-care workers who had contracted the AIDS virus on the job was much too low. "It's certainly much more than eighteen [the figure CDC then used]. It's probably much less than several hundred," he said. Day he said, was part evangelist and part demagogue.

Day announced on 60 Minutes that she was quitting the General—giving up, getting out, exiting the operating room. She'd made the decision months before but had told only a few people.

Along with her dramatic statements, Day's appearance drove home her point. For the operation, she dressed like an astronaut. On her head she placed a thin blue surgical cap, over which she placed a floral paper kerchief, over which she place the Stackhouse space-suit helmet, the one that Dr. Gerberding had laughed off as Day's peculiarity. The round plastic face mask looked like it had been designed by NASA in conjunction with Disneyland. Over the helmet she placed a blue paper hood with a facial opening. She wore an operating-room blue gown, with a microphone taped to her waist. White tubing, like the hose of a vacuum cleaner, trailed from her face mask down her back. On her feet she placed paper booties. Despite her belief that the hospital should supply waterproof footgear, she wore stockings and open-toed high heels underneath her booties. Once she had worn flat shoes during an operation and her staff admonished her that "it ruins your image." She switched back to heels. She'd even done a twenty-two-hour operation in high heels.

In addition to the TV crew, the double team of surgeons—one team for each leg—and the anesthesiologists, Day invited orthopedic surgeon Dr. Don Jewett to measure the aerosols and airborne blood particles. Day was worried that blood-borne particles from HIV-positive patients might be inhaled by anyone in the operating room.

After scrubbing her hands and arms for ten minutes, Day rinsed and fitted two pair of milky white size 6½ latex gloves on her hands. As residents were filing into the operating room, Day was in the hallway speaking to the camera.

With producer, soundman and camera trailing her, Day entered the operating room. She was a vision from *Star Wars*.

One resident cut open the woman's leg. Within minutes he had reached the metal plate. While Day maneuvered a retractor, a forklike instrument that holds the skin, tissue and muscle apart, her resident wielded a screwdriver to remove fourteen two-inch screws from the metal in the woman's leg.

Using a periosteal elevator, they cut off the hard, outer shell and scooped out softer midbone for the bone graft. Blood from the patient's leg gushed down onto the operating-room table and into puddles on the linoleum. It colored the gloves of Day and her team.

Day irrigated the opening, stuffing it with a spongelike towel that quickly bloodied. Just as they were about to put the rod down the woman's leg, Day spotted blood on her paper booties. They had been operating for only half an hour. Day moved to a corner of the room as a resident carried water and yellow soap to her. The *60 Minutes* crew recorded the resident scrubbing Day's big toe. She had to keep her gloved hands clean. Heels and booties put back on, Day returned to the patient.

"We're going to do the reaming in about three minutes," she advised the TV crew, "which is what you asked to see." But the crew was preparing to leave because they had scheduled an appointment with Dr. Bill Schecter, the surgeon (in some ways, Day's opposite), who didn't ask patients to be tested for AIDS before he decided whether to perform surgery. Over Day's polite protestations, they left. As the TV crew talked with Schecter about medical ethics, Day's resident began drilling with the tall reamer. Blood poured and sprayed out of the leg, perfect for the camera that wasn't there. Day wielded a suctioning instrument to help dry out the area. A resident's slate blue gown was splattered with blood.

The resident continued to ream the bone. Although they had not been interviewed by 60 *Minutes*, the residents shared Day's concern. The resident by Day's side, for example, didn't believe physicians should be any more willing to take risks than anyone else. "I don't think there's any amount of money that is worth my life, my patient's life or my staff's life," he said. "This business that physicians are well compensated so they ought to take this risk doesn't apply."

Back during his first year, the surgical resident had used one pair of gloves. But gloves sometimes have microscopic holes, or they tear while in use. As his concern grew, he progressed to two pairs. For this operation, he wore three. To protect his face, he wore a plastic face shield unless he was wearing a space suit. He was not even confident that the space suit completely protected him.

If one of Day's residents was too frightened to operate on an HIV-positive patient she didn't penalize him. Others would perform the operation instead.

"I think things have changed and people are no longer willing to make sacrifices, not only in medicine but in society in general," explained one of Day's residents who was not operating that day. "Everybody's a lot more selfish these days. Doctors are just people like the rest of us, and we've changed along with society, too." The public attitude may be that doctors make a lot more money so more is expected of them. "Society can change but doctors can't, which maybe should be true," he said, "but unfortunately, I don't think it is."

In the operating room, three other residents leaned over the right leg, two over the left. The drill made a high-pitched sound. They worked with vice grips, mallet and pliers. And because Jewett was there to test for the virus in the air, Day took air specimens. Inside their space suits, the surgeons were hot. They talked infrequently and when they did it was with difficulty.

A third resident assisting in the operation resented have so many AIDS patients in surgery. When he was seeing patients in internal medicine, he estimated that 40 percent of his patients had AIDS. "I wanted to see heart attacks, emphysema. I didn't see general medicine." AIDS was interfering in his education. In medical school he'd been assured, "'You'll never get it.' Then you stick yourself and it's a different thing." A lot of his fellow medical students said they'd never practice at the General. As the reamers drilled down, he stood a distance away and spoke: "I don't know how rewarding treating AIDS patients can be because they're terminal. You can't do anything about it," he said, expressing a typical surgical concern. His former girlfriend, now a resident in Iowa, had it easier. "She loves it because they have one AIDS patient in the whole hospital."

Day lifted a clear plastic tube, holding it near the reamer and spray of blood, all part of her personal research into operating-room conditions and AIDS. She had been given fifty-thousand dollars by the orthopedic surgery department at UC Medical School to conduct her own investigation. To prepare for the study, Jewett took a few courses from the American Association of Aerosolization, an organization that focuses on asbestos in the workplace, and he consulted experts. "The air we breathe inside the space suit has been filtered to filter out the virus," Day explained. "We don't know if we can get it that way," which is why Jewett and his machine were testing the blood in the air. A study at Stanford University that simulated operating-room conditions found HIV alive in the air. But no one knew if a person could become infected by breathing that air, Day said.

She held a sterile tube that sucked in the air, wafting it through ten filters. She wanted to know if the particles in the air were small enough to seep through operating room masks.

Two hours into the operation, Day had tiny specks of blood on her plastic face mask. Puddles of blood on the linoleum had swollen into pools. The reaming over, Day and a resident sutured up one leg, a risky procedure that can result in a needle-stick.

Just as she was leaving the operating room, the camera crew returned. "I knew it was going to happen," she said. "You missed the good part."

All Research Is Personal

When news about Q hit, Nurse Vince DeGenova received more than eight hundred calls, a series of uninvited visitors and a drawerful of poignant letters. He'd witnessed the clamor for experimental drugs from desperate men with AIDS before. Nothing prepared him for the response to Q.

Vince was the point man for AIDS drug trials at the General. He had to decide which of the thousands of people wanting to participate in the trials would be selected. The General conducts as many or more AIDS drug tests than anywhere else in the nation. Vince's decision had become the only hope for many people.

Clipped to one of the letters he received were color photos of a boy and girl in baseball uniform:

I am a thirty-nine-year-old heterosexual woman with two children. My husband's condition is further developed than my own. I can definitely feel my body weakening. We are both taking AZT and I am writing to you because I don't know where else to start.

I'm on a crusade to save my family. Mr. DeGenova, this is a reality. My children don't deserve the devastating results of this disease. The ends don't justify the means.

We would like to be included in the test program for Compound Q. If there is any way we can help your study or if there is any way that you can help my family, please do not hesitate to call. . . .

Because participants in drug trials have to live in the Bay Area, the woman and her family were not eligible—they lived out of state.

DeGenova also saved a two-inch stack of cards, held together with a red rubber band. All from the same man, one card arrived for DeGenova every day. The writer wanted his lover to be given Q. One card showed a couple dancing in silvery shadows. Another was an angular man in a tux. Another contained silly sex jokes. Inside each card was a story about the card-writer and his lover. Together, the cards read like a novel. The writer signed each card with such comments as "He's losing his appetite. His weight is dropping."

DeGenova couldn't help but be affected.

Another writer complained:

In May, I wrote you a letter out of despair and urgency. I mailed it through Federal Express. I believed the message of despair would not be a subtle one and I was sure you would have taken at least 5–10 minutes perhaps and would have answered in a positive note. It would have been wonderful to have heard words of encouragement and possibly new treatments "just around the corner."

Well, Mr. DeGenova, thank you so much for your concern. My partner passed away between 4–5 P.M. without ever having any encouraging word from you.

Even the angry letters, DeGenova couldn't throw away. "They think I'm ignoring them," he said wistfully. If only they knew. He'd considered not taking the job. DeGenova, who is a registered nurse and is gay, had watched the distant circle of disease encroach on his life. Initially, "it was always somebody else." Then it became friends. One, then two, then three. A reserved, tidy man, DeGenova would go to a café he hadn't been to in a while and notice that the seats once occupied had emptied. He thought the job at the General might be too much. Then he met Marti Nash, his future boss, known around the office, because of her cuteness and the fact that she's a heterosexual female, as "Gidget does AIDS." She convinced him he would be a very good person for the job because he cared and because he could still be objective "even as emotional as I tend to be at times."

In the early days, everyone was handing him telephone messages. He was calling everyone back—staying until eight or nine every night. Everyone he spoke to was desperate. Every doctor who called had the perfect patient. DeGenova developed a backlog of five hundred unanswered phone messages. If someone wasn't home, he'd call back or leave a simple message: "Tell him Vince called," because he wanted to protect a person's privacy. A lot of times, it took him so long to return the call that people had forgotten who Vince was. Applicants' names were recorded in a red spiral notebook while DeGenova tried to develop a better way.

The phone calls were getting in the way of his central mission. He knew his job was not that of letting people vent their frustrations. He and his boss Nash agreed, "We're here to find answers. We're here to do research." The two decided that "the cause would be better served" by DeGenova's getting people on research trials as fast and efficiently as he could.

Early in his new job, working hard under stressful conditions, he began sleeping sixteen hours a night every Saturday and Sunday. When he awoke, he was still tired.

The doctor gave him the news: He had better get his life in order. He needed to make out his will. DeGenova had severe ARC, the precursor to full-blown AIDS. He was thirty-five.

From a large Italian family, DeGenova is quietly religious. His lover of eight years, a man free of HIV, is a practicing Christian Scientist. The two did not often talk about the nurse's work.

DeGenova told his lover and he telephoned his sister. He couldn't bear telling his parents, knowing how much it would hurt them. He asked his sister to do it. As she cried over the phone she said she couldn't and she wouldn't. Within eighteen hours, all the aunts, uncles and cousins in his close-knit family and his parents, too, heard about DeGenova.

He wrote a will, authorizing has savings to go to pay for college for his two young nephews.

"I think that I am bright and articulate, and I want to live," he said. Recently, he and his lover bought a house, which they are renovating, even though DeGenova knew he might only have a year. He wanted to keep working as long as he could.

To cope with the thousands of requests, DeGenova transferred the names of AIDS patients wanting to participate in drug trials from the red spiral notebook to a computerized database he developed, hoping that the database would not only organize the information better but also shield him from the sorrow he felt for the people who thought he could help. On the computer, he listed applicants' names, telephone numbers, addresses, physicians, their CDC diagnosis and their T cell count. Names were listed according to date of contact. (As the first AIDS research triage in the nation, DeGenova's system has been widely copied.)

But even the computerized data could not always protect him. Late on a Tuesday afternoon, a twenty-eight-year-old German with glasses, short hair and luggage came from the airport. He'd arrived for the cure. The impeccably attired Vince, who looks more like a lawyer than a nurse, was called to the front desk. Under his arm, the man held a rolled-up magazine with a story about Compound Q and a picture of its developer, Dr. McGrath. As DeGenova was starting to talk to the German visitor, the tall, athletic-looking McGrath walked toward them. The German checked his magazine picture with the man coming closer. He called to McGrath and for twenty minutes he begged the scientist to let him try Q. McGrath sent the man back to DeGenova.

DeGenova's heart went out to the German. But DeGenova also knew that was when he had to be most guarded.

The visitor kept telling DeGenova that with German socialized medicine, all the nurse needed to do was give him a prescription and the state would pay. Maybe thirty times, DeGenova told him, "You are not going to be on Q." The visitor heard but would not accept what he was saying. "All you have to do is sign this and I can move here," the German said.

"The patients have already been selected," DeGenova replied.

"No one else can come?" the German asked. "I'm here and I'm willing to take this drug. Why can't you let me take it?" There was desperation in his voice.

DeGenova thought, What makes this man any different from the ones who are in the database? It's a line his boss often used.

Medical reports may make for dry, statistical reading. For DeGenova, all research was personal. The German didn't have much money, so DeGenova brought him home and put him up for the night, instead of finding him a room at the YMCA.

Sometimes the calls, letters and visitors came directly to Dr. Volberding. The hardest to handle were from those people so alone they had nothing to turn to but a name they'd read in the paper. Other times, Volberding received calls from famous people who knew how to work the system. But when an assistant calling for artist Robert Mapplethorpe telephoned in 1989, desperate for Q, Volberding was unimpressed. The assistant pleaded that the world couldn't lose this great man; that he needed the new drug. The artist had less than six months to live. Probably a little blunter than he usually would be, Volberding told the assistant that the artist was too ill to qualify for Q and that it was time for the artist and his associates to recognize what was going on and quit trying to "fly around the world looking for magic cures." Mostly though, Volberding referred such calls to DeGenova.

At times the nurse was lobbied by the political and the powerful. Governors' offices phoned trying to have friends enrolled. One caller offered two hundred thousand dollars for medical research if he could be put on GLQ223. DeGenova told the man the donation would not affect his status and turned down the offer. "However," DeGenova explained, "I did bring it to my boss." Nash backed him up.

Another day, a wheelchair-bound woman from Los Angeles flew up with her mother insisting on seeing DeGenova. He talked to her for several hours, neglecting his work. In her sleep, the Holy Ghost had told her Q was the cure. She believed that DeGenova held the key to her life, if only he could open the door a wedge and let her in.

Her skin was so jaundiced it had turned a tone of tangerine. DeGenova knew just looking at her she wasn't healthy enough to be eligible. She had only 1 T cell left. For her to be included, she would have had to have a lot of lab work, a medical exam, a history, an EKG and a neuropysch exam. DeGenova just said, "It's not going to happen because of logistics." He thought that might be easier for her to accept. It wasn't.

She and her mother stayed all day, refusing to leave at night. "I'm waiting for Vince," she told everyone. Another nurse gave the mother and daughter a taxi voucher and ordered them a cab. She brought them downstairs, but when the cab arrived, they refused it. From which door, they asked, did DeGenova usually leave? When the nurse who had ordered the cab departed, the two were still waiting outside.

Twice a week, DeGenova received a call from a father in Tennessee. The father would say, "I have to talk to Vince. My son is dying." The father wanted his son to be put on the Q trial. The son was too ill and too far away. Times like that, DeGenova had to remind himself of the difference between medical care and research. When DeGenova turned the father down, he told himself, he was denying the son the right to participate in medical research, not denying him medical care or a cure.

The problem with Q was that even though it was only in the earliest, safety tests, everyone approaching DeGenova believed the drug could stop the spread of AIDS. If he believed that Q or any other drug being tested was The Cure he probably couldn't do his job. He had to remind himself that experimental drugs can also kill.

He considered AIDS work as a mosaic. Sometimes the criticism from ACT UP or Project Inform stung him. But everyone, he believed, had a purpose. Whenever he was about to start a drug trial, Vince wrote a summary about the trial's objectives and eligibility and sent his report to Project Inform and other AIDS groups. When calls came from Tulsa and elsewhere asking for information and DeGenova didn't have time, he gave the telephone number for Project Inform.

Sometimes he questioned the rigidity of the regulations. "You get into the whole issue of experimental drugs," DeGenova said. "it's a very confusing issue. You get to the point where you respect what you're doing and the people you're working with but that does not necessarily mean you always have to agree."

One of the patients in DeGenova's database was going blind from CMV (cytomegalovirus) retinitis, one of the opportunistic diseases common to AIDS patients. Having exhausted other remedies, only the experimental drug Foscarnet could save the patient's eyesight. But the General wasn't ready to begin its Foscarnet trial. Believing that the patient should be given the drug, DeGenova told him to call Bay Area Congresswomen Nancy Pelosi and Barbara Boxer and Senator Ted Kennedy.

Suddenly, DeGenova was receiving calls from congressional offices. "Basically they were saying not 'Can you do anything for this guy?' but, 'You will do something for this guy.'"

They wanted to know why the drug trial wasn't ready to begin.

DeGenova went to his boss and said, "'I'm getting these calls from congressional offices'—I didn't necessarily have to say that it might have been because of my instigation that those calls were coming."

The patient was enrolled on Foscarnet. His HIV disease progressed, but he didn't lose his eyesight.

Times like that, DeGenova felt a sense of accomplishment. Other times, he was filled with self-doubt and thought about quitting. Then he recalled that "they don't line up at the doors to work here." A lot of nurses, like a lot of other people, don't like working with AIDS patients. DeGenova knew that many people just think life is good and they don't want to be reminded all the time of tragedies. DeGenova, who cared about what happened, thought, Who would they hire if I left?

Cowboy Medicine

In China, trichosanthin (Compound Q) has been used for two thousand years to treat numerous ailments. Nothing in the Chinese literature suggested it had any toxicity. As part of the Food and Drug Administration–required testing process, lab animals had been infused with GLQ223, Genelabs-produced Q. None had experienced toxic side effects.

Still, McGrath knew that as a plant protein, Q could create a severe allergic reaction. Even recognizing the risks, there was no way he could have anticipated what was to happen.

He didn't need to be reminded of the story of Suramin, used for many years to fight river blindness in Africa and other parasitical diseases. Of all the drugs tested in the early years of AIDS, only Suramin seemed to have specific anti-HIV activity in vitro. Made by Bayer in Germany, it appeared to be reasonably nontoxic, based on studies of people who had taken it.

Volberding and Donald Abrams had flown to the National Institutes of Health in Washington, D.C., to be sure the General could participate in the Suramin clinical trials. They gave the drug to some twenty patients, in amounts equivalent to those used to treat river blindness. By the time Volberding and Abrams detected liver damage in their patients, it was already serious. By Volberding's account, "one or two" of the twenty patients died as a direct result of the drug's toxicity. AIDS activists claimed the death figure was higher. Whatever the number, it became clear that the reaction was not just related to the drug and the dose but to the host as well. Something about AIDS turned Suramin into a toxin.

With Suramin on his mind, McGrath's Q was tested in humans in the late spring of 1989. Reporters cajoled Volberding and McGrath for information. The General's doctors weren't talking.

Meanwhile, rumors were circulating throughout San Francisco that the revolutionary Project Inform had begun underground tests of trichosanthin. Martin Delaney, a prematurely gray, deceptively mild-looking leader, organized the unauthorized Q trial. His brazen move was designed to find fast answers and to circumvent the delays imposed on scientists by the interval before publication of their findings.

While Q tests were under way at the hospital, McGrath was losing his control over the drug forever. A former navy pilot and a nurse whose lover had died of AIDS flew to China to negotiate for ten thousand dollars' worth of trichosanthin for Delaney's experiment. High-tech drugs were beyond their means, but they thought they could get hold of a sufficient amount of Q. American sources had told Project Inform where to find the trichosanthin factor in Shanghai (asked recently if he had been the source, McGrath said he might have been) and which factory workers would be willing to sell. A Chinese gynecologist and her partner, a bus driver, smoothed relations for the Americans, charging twenty-four hundred dollars each for their services. Along the way, Communist Party bureaucrats demanded and received payoffs.

Concerned that AIDS might be unknown or stigmatizing in China, the Americans couched their request for Q in more familiar terms. They said cancer patients would use it. The Chinese responded: You should try it for AIDS.

Under the auspices of the Projects Inform physicians, the Chinese drug was dispensed to cooperative doctors in San Francisco, New York, Los Angeles and Miami. They in turn gave it to forty-two (and later, nine more) severely ill men with AIDS. All of them had signed elaborate release forms, acknowledging that the drug was experimental and might kill them.

The network news shows did stories about Project Inform. The *Wall Street Journal* and the *Los Angeles Times* profiled Delaney. Not long before, he'd been producing videotapes for electronics training. Now he sounded like an activist AIDS doctor. The media glommed on to him as if he were a newly discovered comet in a poorly understood galaxy.

His expertise did little to impress the AIDS establishment, especially the doctors at the General. Delaney and his cowboy clinicians, they argued, lacked outside controls; patients might die needlessly; the pool of eligible volunteers for real drug studies would dry up. They were characterized as pseudoscientists muddying the antiseptic terrain. On *The Today Show*, Volberding argued with Delaney about the underground tests. The AIDS doctor called the underground trial "a disservice to patients." Dr. Jim Kahn, who was conducting the official GLQ223 trial at the General, called it "bad medicine."

Alone among his peers, McGrath befriended the renegades. He didn't want to upset Volberding, a friend from his college days, but McGrath's perspective on drug information differed from that of his colleagues. How could he be possessive about Q when thousands of AIDS patients were dying? When Delaney asked questions, McGrath answered.

The General's human drug trials proceeded on course. At the same time, Project Inform was finding encouraging anecdotal results. After initial flulike symptoms, patients were feeling better, gaining weight, rising from sick beds, painting houses and heading for the ski slopes.

Then, Project Inform ran into trouble. Several men infused with the Chinese Q went into comas. Others couldn't do simple addition and forgot their last names. The reaction was so disastrous, Project Inform doctors feared their trial could be shut down by the feds. The drug that was supposed to be the penicillin of AIDS suddenly looked like poison.

Critics, including the FDA, asserted the trouble was the result of impurities in the Chinese drug. The General's supply of the drug came from Genelabs, which operated under U.S. standards. No one at the General had fallen into a coma. Less well known, however, was the fact that with McGrath's help the Chinese Q, used by Project Inform, had been tested by Genelabs and was found to be pure.

To counter the comas and dementia, Project Inform's unorthodox physicians, Alan Levin, radicalized by the Vietnam War, and Larry Waites, a onetime pediatrician, administered the steroid Decadron in the belief that the problems were brought on by a swelling of the brain. Within twelve hours after the patients had gone into a coma, the new medicine pulled them out of it and their normal mental capacity returned. Shortly afterward, one of the younger patients felt well enough to complain to Delaney that while he'd been comatose his roommate had swiped his stash of marijuana.

Delaney relayed Project Inform's findings to doctors at the General, who were not eager to listen to a former maker of training videos and his free-lance physicians with smuggled drugs. The information was discounted.

The General's Phase I drug trial, or safety test, was proceeding smoothly until August 1989, when it looked as if Q might become another Suramin. Charlie Weaver, a thirty-four-year-old participant in the official hospital drug trials, went into a coma. He'd had the same dosage as his roommate Steve Kubelka. Only Weaver, among all the General's patients infused with Q, became comatose.

For days he remained at the General. Taken off the drug trial, he was placed in the intensive care unit. Reporters had heard about Charlie Weaver, but when they called the General they were told it was "inappropriate" to discuss individual patients. McGrath was not involved in the official trials, but he couldn't help but know what was going on. He felt responsible. The thought of his drug permanently harming anyone shocked him. Maybe Project Inform couldn't prove that Decadron was the antidote to comas. Fine, McGrath thought, there's no proof. But please, God, we should not knock off anybody and we should not have any more comas happen to us.

For months, research nurse DeGenova was haunted by the fact that out of a database of over twelve hundred he had selected Charlie Weaver. Every day Weaver was in the ICU, DeGenova visited. He held Weaver's hand and whispered in his ear, "Charlie, just keep fighting. Please keep fighting." DeGenova felt awful. He had been trying to help people with AIDS and here was someone harmed, he thought, by his effort.

In desperation, Weaver's roommate Kubelka called Project Inform's doctors, beseeching them to intervene. Delaney, in turn, wrote a letter to the FDA's antiviral drug department, complaining about the treatment of Charlie Weaver. That the steroid Decadron should be administrated to a comatose patient, Delaney wrote, "would be obvious to most first-year residents for any general brain encephalopathy."

One of the Project Inform physicians momentarily considered kidnapping Charlie Weaver and taking over his care. Instantly the politically astute Delaney vetoed it. He thought Weaver had been comatose for so long that he might have suffered permanent brain damage. If Project Inform took over his care, the group could be blamed for his deteriorated condition.

In late August 1989, while Weaver lay in a coma, Chinese scientists flew into San Francisco to talk to Project Inform's doctors. They were worried, they said, about the bad reputation Q was developing and how that might reflect on their nation. They seemed unaware that their country's image had been ruined only a few weeks before by the massacre at Tiananmen Square. (Before they arrived, Delaney had worried that the Chinese might have an alternative motive: defection.) At their first meeting, the scientists sipped red cans of Coca-Cola Classic while Project Inform doctors questioned them about the side effects of the ancient drug. The Chinese had their own, more formal agenda. The Chinese word for trichosanthin, they began, means "heaven flower powder." Delaney and the Project Inform physicians smiled. They were not terribly interested in literal translations. They wanted to cut to the controversy.

"There is currently a belief [your drug] is not pure," a Project Inform doctor warned.

"This good man will put out the truth," said Dr. Gua-Qiang Lin, deputy director of the Shanghai Institute of Organic Chemistry, reaching over to pat the knee of an alternative-press reporter wearing a neon-green shirt, purple band around his ponytail and a collection of earrings.

The Chinese were anxious to formalize the drug sales. One of their scientists complained that desperate AIDS patients were calling him at his home.

After repeated questions, the Chinese physicians said they had never experienced comas or dementia with Q. This was important. It probably meant that the toxic reaction was the result of AIDS.

Doctors at Project Inform established that Q had only harmed the sickest patients: those with AIDS-related brain damage prior to taking the drug and with fewer than one hundred T cells left. The General's doctors did a scan of Weaver's brain and a spinal tap. In neither case did they find any indication of brain swelling, which would have led them to consider administering steroids. But after they had tried everything else they could think of, Weaver was given Decadron. About a week later he emerged from his coma, but he never fully recovered.

After that, both the General and Project Inform began excluding patients with T cell counts below one hundred from the trials.

Charlie Weaver had walked into the General. He'd looked and sounded healthy. But in fact, he had only twenty of the disease-fighting T cells left.

The day Weaver was discharged from the General to go to another hospital for rehabilitation, Nurse DeGenova came to say goodbye. Weaver was sitting in a chair, still mentally disabled. His roommate was there to pick him up.

"Why didn't you listen?" Kubelka asked DeGenova.

"Why didn't you know what was going on in the underground trial?"

The decision had not been DeGenova's to make. He had been the recruiting nurse, not the physician.

"We are in phase one of the drug trial [in which safety is determined]," DeGenova explained. He told Weaver's roommate the doctors at the General didn't even know if Project Inform was dispensing the same drug, if they were treating patients at the same stage in their illness, or what dosage they were dispensing.

If he understood the argument, Weaver said nothing. When he rose to leave, the patient threw his arms out toward the nurse who had let him join the Q trial. Weaver gave him a kiss goodbye. The sweet farwell eased the pain DeGenova felt. But he wished he had never put Charlie Weaver on the list to test GLQ223.

Charlie Weaver never returned to San Francisco General. He died several months later in Palm Springs—where he and Kubelka had gone to recover—of an AIDS-related infection.

Money, Politics and Turf

Nearly two years had passed and Jane Doe still hadn't received any money from the city. She wanted no more than four people in the city attorney's office and its retirement office to know her identity. But the city, represented by deputy city attorney Dan Maguire, refused to alter its policies to suit someone infected with HIV. The city contended that its regular procedures would be adequate to protect Jane Doe, although it would not specify how many people needed to know her true name.

Despite the fact that the issue was unresolved, it took a peculiar case of civic chutzpah to schedule a deposition for Jane Doe. Did the city really expect a woman unwilling to reveal her name to show up for questioning? If she wouldn't tell them her true name, did they expect her to divulge her personal history during a deposition?

Feisty attorney Patricia Hastings and Jane Doe hatched a plan. Jane Doe asked her hospital friends for help, and they in turn asked others. Hastings went to ACT UP and told its members, "There's this little straight kid from New York who has no risk factors. She's out there fighting for every gay man on the street."

When, at the last minute, the deposition was canceled, the plan still went into effect.

"Are you here to see me?" inquired deputy city attorney Maguire when Jane Doe appeared at his office.

"I believe you have an appointment at nine," Jane Doe responded.

"Do you mean the deposition?"

"Yes."

"The deposition has been canceled."

"Yes," the nurse said, "But I believe you still have that slot open. There are several of us who'd like to speak to you."

She left the office and went to the staging area, returning with some thirty people wearing Jane Doe name tags. Into Maguire's office came nurses in their whites, one AIDS nurse with her twins in a baby carriage, TV reporters and cameramen.

"We know you wanted to depose Jane Doe. We're here to tell you we are all Jane Doe and you can ask us anything you'd like," said San Francisco General nurse Bill Walker. What transpired, of course, was that the nurses and activists ended up interrogating the civil servant. For an hour and a half they questioned his motives and his inactivity. And the real Jane Doe got to look him in the eye without feeling vulnerable. She was just one person in an angry crowd. Normally uncomfortable speaking in public, courage came to her. She straightened up, looked straight at Maguire and said: "We have it from Jane Doe's lawyer that you have had verification for eighteen months from Dr. Julie Gerberding because she wrote a letter almost immediately. Then she sent another this past spring that Jane Doe indeed was a nurse working with people with AIDS, that she stuck herself with a needle from an HIV-positive person, that she developed a febrile illness, that she was tested prior to the illness and was negative, that she was found to be positive by multiple tests, that you have had everything you needed except her name." As she spoke, her eyes hardened. The TV cameras zoomed in. Her anger and the simplicity of her statement worked.

Finally, a woman stood up and said, "Are you telling me you don't believe Dr. Julie Gerberding? Dr. Gerberding says Jane Doe's a city employee. Phil Sowa [the hospital's administrator] says she's a city employee. Maybe you don't believe Phil Sowa is a city worker. Maybe you don't believe anything, Mr. Maguire. What do you believe? Do you believe the name your mother gave you?"

When it was over, the people from ACT UP approached the real Jane Doe, not knowing she was *the* Jane Doe. "You're hot," they said. "You ought to join." Despite her effervescence, Jane Doe did not seek confrontation. She declined their invitation. But there was nothing like fighting for herself. At that moment, she was soaring.

Within days, the city succumbed. After months of telling Jane Doe that it could not possibly comply with her request, deputy city attorney Maguire proposed a settlement that was better than any Jane Doe had proposed. No more than four people would ever know her true identity: one in the city attorney's office and one in the workers' compensation division, and, in case of emergency—such as determining whether or not Jane Doe had been properly paid—then the city attorney and Clare Murphy, manager of the retirement board, would be informed.

"It is kind of a sobering joy, like when a war ends and you count the casualties," Jane Doe told the *Chronicle*. "It was about numbers and money and politics and egos and turf. It wasn't about a human being. If it had been one of their siblings or lovers or daughters, things would have moved differently."

All along the city had worried about Jane Doe's case establishing a precedent. When it was over, city officials claimed that it hadn't.

"Honey," said attorney Hastings, "it walks like a precedent. It talks like a precedent. It even quacks like a precedent. They can call it whatever they want." Precedent was important. Every month, approximately forty-five hospital employees—doctors, nurses, gardeners, janitors and others—were using the needle-stick hotline to report being exposed to patient blood or body fluid. One out of every three hundred and thirty-three people at the hospital seriously exposed to the HIV virus through their work was expected to convert. The hospital estimated that one employee every five years would contract the virus on the job.

The following week, the Service Employees International Union Local 790, the nurses' union, won a clause in it's contract that not more than four people in city government would be informed if a nurse became HIV positive on the job. Jane Doe's right to confidentiality had been extended to others. She wanted to frame the clause like an award.

After the agreement was reached, Attorney Maguire finally had his chance to depose Jane Doe. An informal event, without a stenographer, he met Jane Doe and Hastings in the conference room of Hastings's law firm.

The city already had been informed by Gerberding, head of the health-care workers study at San Francisco General, that blood-to-blood contact was far more infective than sexual transmission. Hastings told Jane Doe she needn't answer questions about her sex life. "I personally think her sex life has nothing to do with it," Hastings explained. "If they want to hear about somebody's sex life, I'll be happy to tell them about mine."

As they waited for Maguire, Jane Doe was shaking with rage. How was she going to speak to this person? She was so angry with him and everyone he represented. When he arrived, however, her anger subsided. In the conference room, her turf and that of her lawyer's, he was no longer a threatening presence.

Maguire asked Jane Doe for a list of all her physicians, including those in nursing school. He needed to know every place she'd worked. She delighted in telling him that when she came to San Francisco she had worked out of a registry, going to seven hospitals. Ha, she thought, how was he going to trace that? He asked about every hospital she'd worked in while on rotation in nursing school. He asked about the AIDS patient whose blood had infected Jane Doe. She didn't remember his name. He asked for a blood-bank card, given when someone donates blood. He wanted her blood-bank records. Hastings's patience began waning. She had little tolerance for "this petty bureaucratic bullshit when my people are dying in droves." But in the conference room, she stayed cool. Jane Doe was asked to describe the details of the accident, the key players, the tests, the illness. Maguire asked if Jane Doe had ever used IV drugs. (The answer was no.) He asked about her sex life, her sexual history. Had she ever been with anyone who had been with anyone at risk? To Jane Doe it felt like a "lukewarm rape trial."

"To tell you the truth, Mr. Maguire, I think this whole deposition is unnecessary," Jane Doe replied. "It's icing on the cake. You have all the information you need and you have had all the information you needed for over a year."

Hastings suggested a question Maguire might ask that would not offend Jane Doe or herself. So he asked, "As a medical health professional, to your knowledge was there any other way you could have contracted the disease?"

"No."

When they'd been battling the bureaucrats, Jane Doe didn't have to think about the virus all the time. Hastings had made the fight easier, she had kept the city from directly hassling her. Together, they made it easier for whoever would come after her. Ultimately though, Hastings felt powerless because the truth was that, "We can't do anything about her situation. And we can't stop the next one." Hastings said she became wrapped up in the legalities of it "because I can't fucking stand to deal with the fact that I can't do anything."

Shortly after the city agreed to the anonymity clause, Jane Doe and her attorney walked home together. "You know, Trish," Jane Doe said, "basically, we've won. They've agreed to everything. We basically got what we wanted and now I have to look and say, 'I've still got this virus.'"

Iron Pills

"Oh, my neck hurts. Do I have AIDS?"

Melissa Bartick had no easy answers. Just questions. A senior medical student at the University of California Medical School at San Francisco, she was doing her rotation at a health clinic affiliated with the General in the city's predominantly black neighborhood of Bayview Hunters Point. Melissa was Jane Doe's contemporary, although the two had never met. Medical students couldn't help but be affected by Jane Doe or, for that matter, by Dr. Day. They confronted the issues in every ward and clinic and would have to decide if they wanted to practice in urban settings or in safer locations.

The first time Melissa had seen the man for his checkup he'd indicated he had no risk factors for AIDS. Reassuringly, she'd told him he probably didn't have to worry, but she warned him about the risks of contracting the disease from heterosexual sex. The questions were the same this time. The answers varied. Melissa already knew that some minority men who engaged in homosexual sex did not consider themselves gay or bisexual. This time she again asked about his sexual orientation.

"I'm straight."

Often, declaratory sentences can be more complex than they seem.

"Do you ever have sex with men?"

"Sort of."

On this, his second visit to the Southeast Health Clinic, he mentioned for the first time his weight loss, crack use and "sort of" gay sex. And he complained of undefined ailments. Melissa expressed concern.

"My health just isn't right," the patient said. "Can I have iron pills?"

If only AIDS were that easy. She told him about the AIDS test.

"How much blood do you have to take?"

"Your body makes new blood all the time," she told him.

"Can you prescribe iron pills?"

When high on crack, he sometimes forgot to eat. She suggested that if he stopped doing crack his health might improve. He said he wanted to gain weight. Melissa gave him a diet chart, circling the "Do Not Eat" section and told him that's what he should eat—ice cream, whole milk.

"Some days I go out every day, hustling." The meaning of the word *hustle* hung ambiguously in the small examining room. "I might smoke in a whole day about thirty, forty dollars. I got in the habit of standing out in the street. I was wearing myself down. . . . My cousin said, 'I think you went crazy.' Nobody has control over your mind when you use that stuff. Everybody's out there for the first hit. I know it's a false feeling."

His face was almond shaped. Serious eyes looked down on a prominent nose. He seemed far older than his twenty years. On a play-ball kind of day, he wore a long-sleeved jersey and a button-down shirt and jacket.

Melissa paused to sniffle—her sixth cold of the year. She'd also sustained two flus. With the daily stress, she was wearing herself down. She asked if he'd taken her advice and sought help for his crack addiction at Glide Memorial Church, a downtown church that offered help to societal rejects.

"I haven't looked into that yet."

Melissa came across not as an authority figure but more as a peer/friend. She was wearing a pink-and-gray checked cotton shirt and dark pants. Her long brown hair swept along the sides of her head and was held in back by a sensible, schoolgirl red barrette. Her hair flowed down her right shoulder. The stethoscope hung down the left. She leaned forward on her metal swivel chair and in a soft voice urged her patient to action. He promised to go to the downtown church for drug help.

"When?" she asked.

"Not yet."

Her decency and dedication trailed her like a shadow. Into a wicker basket at the front desk, she had poured Trojan condoms with little messages: DON'T LET AIDS GET YOU! TAKE ONE. TAKE SOME. OR ASK YOUR DOCTOR OR NURSE FOR MORE! Friendly coworkers chided her— either for her naïveté or her earnestness. But regularly the basket needed to be replenished.

In the spring of 1990, she drew up two flyers, one about pregnancy and crack, the other about crack, pregnancy and AIDS. Her posters, written in English and Spanish, were distributed at the General and to health clinics in the city. One poster read: "Yo, Women! How can using CRACK and alcohol give AIDS to you and your baby?" AIDS, it explained, was a sexually transmitted disease. "You may be too high or too drunk to think of using condoms! You cannot tell who has the virus even if they seem clean!"

Some time after that when Melissa was attending a gathering of female crack addicts at Glide Memorial Church, one of the women said, "Every time I think about using, I just look at this poster." Melissa looked at the wall and taped to it was her flyer. Melissa was pleased; she had reached someone.

She thought prevention was so much cheaper, less painful. And in her small way, she liked to educate.

Having grown up in the era of busing, Melissa remembered many of her white friends being pulled out of Alexandria, Virginia, schools in the sixth grade by their parents. By the time she reached high school, her class was 48 percent black, 42 percent white. The rest were "mostly Iranian and Southeast Asian refugees." Most of the blacks lived in the projects; not many of the whites did. The inequity of it gnawed at her. She found a relatively homogeneous student body at the University of Virginia and missed being around different ethnic groups. Medicine was a way of getting back to them and it was a way of helping. In the beginning, AIDS was just another way to help and to explore the inequities she saw.

When she worked in 5A, the AIDS Ward at San Francisco General, her patients at times were frighteningly well informed. Once, she asked a man to describe his chief complaint: "I was just diagnosed with toxo and my Compazine lowered my seizure threshold and I had a grand mal tonic-clonic seizure." Here at Southeast, her population was disenfranchised and her patient thought he could stave off death with an iron pill.

"Hopefully, if I don't have AIDS maybe I'll start feeling better," the patient said. She talked about the AIDS antibody test and told him they were developing new drugs all the time.

"Do you know what AZT is?"

"It's a lotion they give to AIDS patients to get rid of the bumps on their faces," he said.

She taught him about the drug and told him not to worry about his test results being disclosed. They'd go in an envelope in the back of his medical chart. "They don't send it out to insurance companies. They make every effort to protect your privacy." (Within months, she would think that statement naïve. If insurance companies want to find out, she thought they could. Almost surely, the patient didn't have any insurance anyway.)

"If you're positive, it does not mean you're going to die tomorrow," she counseled. "It can be more than five years. It can also be less than that," she said. (The average latency period, from contracting the virus to onset of AIDS, is ten years.) And she told him that even if his test results were negative, he already could be carrying the disease. "If you've been exposed in the last six months, it may not show up on the test," she said.

He nodded, adding, "On the news they said it can take up to three years to find it if you have the virus."

That's the thing about AIDS. It was so new that more information spurted out daily. Even this patient, with his rudimentary knowledge, knew more about the lead time for antibodies than the medical student did.

During her entire medical-school career, Melissa recalled having only one or two lectures entirely on AIDS, but those were about viral structure, nothing that might help an inexperienced clinician at the General. When she entered medical school in 1984, not much was known about the new disease. Melissa spent her first three years at the University of California at Berkeley in a special class of twelve, before going over to UC Medical School in San Francisco. She recalled one colloquy in which a person with AIDS came to speak. It was the first time she'd ever seen anyone with AIDS. Another time, a medical student told a lecturer, "I've gone to six funerals already. When is it going to end?" Now, she just walked down her block in San Francisco's Castro district and saw "men with purple spots on their faces, young men in wheelchairs or walking with canes." Sometimes she passed men in their twenties with oxygen tanks with nasal cannula that allowed them to breathe. Some of what Melissa learned about the disease she picked up from fellow students. Most of what she knew, she learned at the General. "It feels like I'm learning what I need to know about it," she explained during a peanut-butter-and-jelly lunch at the clinic. Her copy of *The Medical Management of AIDS*, edited by Paul Volberding and Merle Sande, was the only book she owned devoted to a single disease. "And it's one of my most used books."

With the AIDS patients as well as the others at Southeast Health Clinic, Melissa felt she had established a symbiotic relationship. She tended to them while they helped her better understand the complicated issues behind becoming an IV drug user or a homeless person or ignoring the precautions against contracting AIDS.

Periodically Melissa tried to telephone another patient about his AIDS test. He'd pulled a muscle in his leg and came to her thinking it meant he had AIDS. His twenty-six-year-old brother had died of AIDS two years before, having kept his homosexuality hidden. At twenty-five, this patient figured he was dying, too. Melissa suggested he be tested. He consented, but said if he was positive he would kill himself "right there." Melissa was worried. The patient was supposed to pick up his results at the General.

She telephoned the patient's girlfriend. He no longer lived there. The girlfriend had her own medical problems she wanted to share with Melissa. The medical student seized the opportunity: "Make sure he uses a condom. You never know where he's been."

The girlfriend said no problem. Her boyfriend had already received his AIDS test results and assured her he was negative. Then she told Melissa that sometimes he lied.

"Please pass along the message that he should be careful," Melissa advised. "He still needs some counseling. He still doesn't understand what it means." The girlfriend provided two other telephone numbers.

Melissa dialed a residential hotel. She gave his room number. The woman who answered the hotel phone said no one was going to go to his room.

"This is his doctor's office calling. It's really important," Melissa said.

"I don't care who this is," said the woman. *Click.*

She tried the next number and said it was Dr. Bartick calling. Since she was still a medical student, Melissa didn't like to call herself a doctor but just then she needed the clout. He wasn't there either.

She had to go back to her other patients. Melissa saw a robust woman with a shopping list of ailments. When asked, "Are you allergic to anything?" the woman didn't hesitate: "My ex-husband and dust."

Schoolchildren had booby-trapped the classroom door for the principal, who had cut their recess short. The patient, then working in the classroom, walked in first. A table toppled onto her hand, severely injuring it.

Melissa was painstakingly thorough and attentive with the patient although she kept thinking about the man who wanted to kill himself if he had the AIDS virus. A clinic such as this one had been jammed with patients before AIDS intruded. Now, Melissa had to squeeze those patients in.

When Melissa finished her examination, she walked past the waiting room on her way to the nursing station. "Oh, my stars!" she said on discovering a white-haired grandmother and shy little boy in the waiting room. Melissa had been wanting to see the boy, but each time they made an appointment, the boy and his grandmother failed to show. This time they came unexpectedly. They would have to wait.

Melissa spotted the patient she'd been trying to reach by phone: He was walking the hallways, looking for her. His girlfriend had tracked him down and sent him to Melissa.

"My bus transfer is up at two-thirty," he said at ten to three.

"Don't worry about it," Melissa said.

Next, he volunteered that he hadn't picked up his test results "because I didn't have transportation." And even if he had had transportation, he'd lost his identification paper. Conducted anonymously, the General would only give him his test results if he presented his code number.

He seemed more concerned about the bus transfer than about his test results. Melissa pushed ahead: "Are you worried about what the results are going to be?"

"Yeah."

Melissa said she'd give him his identification number again. Then she asked him to go over with her the various ways someone can contract AIDS.

Tall, with a long face and slow lisp, he explained, "By having sex with another woman who's got it. By catching different kinds of disease. You can get AIDS by germs. I don't know," he said, legs swinging nervously from the exam table.

Melissa asked how he thought he could have contracted AIDS.

"I must have gotten it from my brother."

She asked if he'd had sex with his brother or shared a needle with him. The patient said he hadn't.

"Then if you have AIDS, you didn't get it from him."

When Melissa first met the patient, he had come into the clinic with the worst case of gonorrhea she'd ever seen. He'd been angry with his girlfriend and in spite, had gone to bed with a woman who had a venereal disease.

Yet he was telling Melissa, "I'm a typical man. I don't just go out with any woman. I don't fool around. I don't even have sex with my old lady anymore. All we do is talk on the phone."

"You had sex with the other woman. That's how you got gonorrhea," Melissa reminded him.

"Hmm. Hmm."

The patient said he would be cautious with his girlfriend. "If I be knowing her, I'll use condos [sic]," he promised. A seeming sweetness was sewn into his ignorance. "If I get AIDS I would let her know. I wouldn't put her life before me," he said. "I would use a condom."

If he was HIV positive, he might already have given her the virus.

Melissa wanted him to understand the risks. "If you have sex with someone who uses needles, you can get it," she said.

"I see."

"I don't mess around with gay men," he offered.

"AIDS is everywhere," Melissa said, leaning in toward her patient. "Anyone can get it."

Yin and Yang

J. B. Molaghan surged down the hallway. His dirty-blond hair in a sharp buzz, his body taut from six-day-a-week workouts, he resembled a gymnast on his way to a Wheaties commercial. On this Thursday morning, he rounded the corner of Ward 86, the AIDS outpatient unit, stopping by the mini–intensive care unit for outpatients too ill to leave.

"You look so much better than last week," J.B. chirped. "You don't look as pale. Your lips are pink." But for the thatch of puffy brown hair, the patient looked nearly lifeless. His beard was neatly trimmed. He wore a pair of gold-rimmed glasses. Tucked under the sheets and a thermal blanket, his wiry body resembled a pencil wrapped in blue cloth. As the two talked, J.B. stroked the patient's hair.

With this, his third bout of pneumonia, the patient was told he would need a blood transfusion the next day.

"If you stop breathing, would you want to be resuscitated?" J.B. asked.

"Gee. That's a heavy question."

"We have to write it on your chart," he gently explained.

"I haven't finished making my will so I guess I would say yes," the patient said. "What's your advice?"

"If there are things you want to take care of. . . ." J.B. said, speaking softly to the wasted young man with the look of an old one.

They talked about how the patient might feel being hooked up to a machine. Generally, J.B. said soothingly, blood transfusions are uneventful. Sometimes, though, problems arise.

"There are times in people's lives when they want to be resuscitated," J.B. said. "And there are times in their lives when they don't. Now," he said, "your will to live is quite strong."

Down the hallway, in front of the busy nursing station, the lover of another patient was screaming at the nurses. J.B., the head nurse of Ward 86, was summoned. The handsome, dark-haired man with well-defined features and sweat beads peeling down his forehead was rambling, crying and shouting at the nurses: "I'm a highly intelligent person! No one ever acknowledges that. I'm watching the man I care about die! Who cares about the caregiver?" He couldn't figure out how to open the wheelchair for his sick lover. As he fiddled with the levers, he told J.B. that he knew one of the receptionists hated him. "Her life isn't going to end when David dies. I love David more than anyone on the face of the earth," he said, burying his head in J.B.'s chest.

"I have ARC," he blurted out. "I apologize for the emotional outburst. I'd just love to be in one [research] study before I croak. How do I get David out?"

"There's a ramp," J.B. said calmly.

Every day it was different and every day it was the same. Death, death and more death. To the uninitiated, 86 seemed like a vault of depression. Yet despite the horror, the chaos, the constant crises and the warlike environment, those who work there found the atmosphere "quite wonderful." As long as there was an epidemic, many Ward 86 nurses felt they wouldn't want to be anywhere else.

J.B. wore turquoise or magenta shirts to work, as if he were punching death in the jaw. No nurse on the ward wore white, because J.B. said, patients were vulnerable enough; they didn't need to be intimidated. He and the other nurses asked patients to call them by their first names. On the unit, the barrier between health-care professional and patient often was smudged. At times, the ebullient J.B. could be observed bounding down the hallway singing "Working My Way Back to You Babe" and other pop rock tunes. Yet he'd cared for hundreds of patients from diagnosis to death. Like a trampoline artist, for every downward pull, his effervescent character seemed to somersault above it.

That wasn't always so. The early years were so painful that J.B. called in sick a lot and he was also drinking too much. (He quit drinking years ago, adopting a healthier life-style and better means of coping through exercise and group sports.) He dreaded telling people where he worked. At a dinner party, he'd skip the subject because all anyone would say was, "That's nice. What do you think of the 49ers?"

The hardest part was calculating the right distance to keep between himself and his patients. The nurses on Ward 86 were professional but they were more than that. Gently and quietly, they provided more than physical care for their patients. J.B. wanted to be close, but he couldn't hurt all the time. He didn't want to become used to people dying and being in pain. He wanted to be touched by it. Over time he found the right equation. For the patients to whom he felt binding ties, J.B. made house calls long after they'd quit coming to clinic. For them, as much as for himself, he wanted to be there for their dying. In time he got used to death, although it was nothing he was very proud of.

As J.B. maintained an uncanny cheeriness about the ward, Nurse Gary Carr, supervisor of nurse practitioners for 86, suffered. He'd counted ninety-four of his patients on the AIDS quilt. Chubby, with curly red hair and a singsong sadness to his New York accent, he seemed to soak up the sorrow on the ward. When he had begun working with AIDS patients years ago, he had read a lot of books about the Holocaust. They made him appreciate dignity in death and feel that gay men were not alone.

In his cubicle, Gary posted the Hebrew Prayer for the Dead, given to him by the family of a patient, and an obituary of Neil, a patient he'd loved ("published poet, cat breeder, rapscallion. . . . taught yoga to people with AIDS. . . ."). Even in sorrow, levity cropped up. On Gary's desk sat a white, Styrofoam cup used by Elizabeth Taylor when she had visited 5A. The cup is encased in a clear plastic dome. Gary denied grabbing for the souvenir. The nurses on 5A gave it to him, he explained.

Gary and J.B. are the yin and yang of Ward 86. Gary is Jewish and full of pathos. J.B. is Irish Catholic. When they speak, both men sprinkle their sentences with Yiddishisms. And when they recount their history, political activism and a family death are a part of both.

J.B. grew up near Boston, one of six kids in a family known for having a good time. His parents, J.B. recalled, were always busy with all of them, never busy with just one. At the dinner table there was not a lot of eye contact. When J.B.'s father was diagnosed with cancer, his son was sent to live with an older sister. The family did not talk about death; they didn't want the kids to suffer. His father died at age forty-two.

His senior year of high school, J.B. skipped eighty-nine days of class, eventually dropping out to join antiwar protesters in Harvard Square. Later he earned a high-school equivalency degree, went on to college and to graduate from the Harvard Medical School Nurse Practitioner Program at Massachusetts General Hospital.

Gary had been politicized by the Vietnam War and, like J.B., he came to believe that by his actions he could make a difference. Working days at an ad agency in 1973, he began volunteering evenings at St. Mark's clinic, which devoted one night to lesbians with an all-lesbian staff, two nights to gay men with an all-gay male staff and two nights for anyone, with a mixed staff.

When Gary's grandmother died at ninety-two, she was surrounded by her children, grandchildren and great-grandchildren. People wailed. They carried on. That, Gary thought, was about as good as death got.

By contrast, one of his aunts tried to keep her cancer a secret from the family, claiming she was suffering from arthritis. He knew and she knew, but neither could say. She died surrounded by an air of embarrassment. Since then, Gary had often thought about his aunt, especially when he had had to level with a patient. "Better I should say [the truth] than they should have to die like my aunt, surrounded by a lie."

"Don't be afraid to say 'AIDS,'" Volberding told him on his first day working with the disease. Since then, Gary has told dozens of people they have AIDS. Afterward he sometimes has had to lock himself in the bathroom and cry.

Still, given the circumstances, he wouldn't want to be anywhere else. When he was younger, he worked at Mount Sinai Hospital in New York, and a lot of the time he spent "being a maid." The hospital, he felt, was designed to suit the doctors, not the patients or the staff. And when he told older people he was a registered nurse (he later became a nurse practitioner), they assumed his job was mostly making beds. At

Bellevue in New York, where he'd also worked, and at the General, he was given independence. When he and J.B. started at the clinic in 1983, they followed Volberding and Abrams around for a while, then were given their own patients.

To keep them up to date about the disease, J.B. attended the Thursday-morning meetings to discuss new, unusual cases.

On this Thursday they discussed the case of a nine-year-old girl who'd stepped on her uncle's needle from an AIDS drug injection. The doctors at the General immediately had offered AZT for the little girl, which is recommended for health-care workers with needle-sticks. The family declined. They talked about several men diagnosed with toxoplasmosis without having had PCP, the AIDS pneumonia. For most HIV-positive patients, PCP was the first opportunistic infection. Suddenly the hospital was finding a run of toxo patients. As they talked, the thirty-something doctors and assorted nurses sipped coffee and ate bagels. When the meeting ended, J.B. called out, "Let's be careful out there."

Often, patients are as informed as the nurses and doctors, tossing medical journals at them and asking for a reaction.

Among the patients J.B. saw that afternoon was an MIT scholarship student in San Francisco for the summer. The student planned to fly from Boston once a month to see J.B. It was, he said, cheaper to pay the airfare than to pay for Massachusetts medical care. Besides, he liked the acupuncture (not at Ward 86), massage and San Francisco atmosphere. An intense, compact man, the patient asked J.B. his views on the new drug DDI, on Compound Q and on persantine. "I've read it can increase the effectiveness of AZT," the patient said.

In the waiting room, lean men sat in angular positions. With blank expressions, they watched cartoons on TV, read and ate square chocolate chip cookies, baked by Mary Rathbun, the volunteer patron saint of Ward 86.

J.B. examined Jerry, a patient coming near the end. He had uncontrollable diarrhea, thrush, Kaposi's sarcoma and numbness in his legs. He lived in a third-floor walk-up. His talk was slowed; his conversation coherent. His graceful hands arched through the air of the exam room as he spoke. "This old lady isn't what she used to be," he said, patting his lap, on which he'd placed a black leather jacket that once fit. When his friends were told they had AIDS they stayed inside for weeks, seeing no one. Some fought against it. Jerry would go along for the ride. He used to worry about medical bills. Not anymore. They weren't worth getting upset about.

Another patient with occasional depression was overly optimistic during the exam. Richard had visited his twenty-five-year-old younger brother in Florida when the brother was dying of AIDS. The younger sibling, "a gorgeous little kid," looked like an old man on his deathbed. Richard found the awful image of his baby brother "disgusting." Richard promptly went home, stuffed pills down his throat, drank alcohol, turned on the oven and slashed his wrists. He lived. Richard no longer believed he'd die the way his little brother had, and, in a note of great optimism, he asked J.B. to find him a therapist.

Between the deaths of his patients, J.B. saw the hyphens of life. When things worked, J.B. could treat patients and give them months of relative health. John, his next patient, was convinced that J.B. could mend whatever was broken. When John came down with PCP, J.B. made him well again; when John became demented and went to Hollywood, convinced he was going to appear on a game show, J.B. had an AIDS group find him in a park where he was encamped and fly him home. J.B. put him on AZT, which improved the dementia. But when J.B. couldn't fix everything, and he knew he couldn't, John became angry. Times like that, J.B. and Gary had to remind themselves of their limitations. And when the anger capsized, as it sometimes did, they reminded themselves that they hadn't given the patient AIDS.

Increasingly, more and more patients were IV drugs users, some of them full of fury and misunderstanding; many of them street smart and manipulative. Sometimes J.B. had to quell fights; more and more often, security guards had to be called. Once, a streetwise AIDS patient, believed to be under the influence of drugs, had threatened to come after the nurses with his gun.

For J.B. and Gary, the stress of patient care was interspersed with other tasks. J.B. fielded calls almost every day from nurses in Florida, Montana, upstate New York, and elsewhere. Patronizingly, they'd tell him, "You're the experts. We don't have the facilities. . . ." They wanted to slough off their AIDS patients. So J.B. would respond, "Do you have an X-ray machine? Do you have a needle?" And he'd talk them through AIDS care. Many times he spoke about his experiences to social workers, doctors and nurses at conferences in Honolulu, Atlanta, Denver, Boston, Rochester and St. Louis. And when TV cameramen showed up to do AIDS stories, J.B. often was trotted out as the articulate, charismatic spokesman.

His first major media encounter occurred in 1985 when, J.B. said, "AIDS was big and I was naïve." Mark Segars, a quiet, shy, cowboy type was flying home to Atlanta to say goodbye to the family he hadn't seen in fifteen years. J.B. called customer service at Delta Airlines to make arrangements for Mark to bring oxygen onto the plane, just in case he needed it. Although he had the oxygen with him, Segars never used it on his flight to Atlanta. When he was ready to return home, Mark was told that he could not fly, allegedly because he would require frequent supervision. With the approval of the very private Mark, J.B. telephoned Mobilization Against AIDS, an advocacy group. All Mark wanted to do was to come home to his friends to prepare to die. In the Bible Belt, some news accounts said Mark was oozing with sores. In the Bay Area, doctors and nurses went on the air to say no one could contract AIDS from an airline seat. Eastern and TWA offered to fly Mark home. On his return flight, Mark was met by a limo on the runway. J.B. and friends brought champagne for the ride. J.B. climbed onto the plane to bring his patient out. With J.B.'s help, Mark had set a precedent for airline travel. Four weeks after he'd flown home on TWA, Mark died.

Gary's encounters tended to be more in-house. When a group of African doctors visited the General, Gary and Dr. Michael Clement, the supervising doctor on 86, gave an informal talk in a hospital auditorium, with Gary translating from French. Clement spoke optimistically about AZT—not a cure, he said, but a drug that "hopefully will buy us time to find a cure." At the time, AZT cost about six thousand to eight thousand dollars per patient each year. What he didn't say was that he was embarrassed to be discussing AZT because he knew, at those prices, the drug was irrelevant to what was happening in Africa.

"Do we recommend vitamins?" Gary asked, translating a question.

"We encourage our patients in whatever way is good for them, to maintain good nutrition; not to lose weight," he said diplomatically. A nutritionist is available to clinic patients two days a week, he said.

"What about vitamins?" someone else asked again.

"I don't give them vitamins," he said.

Another doctor pursued the question.

"Vitamins don't reverse the process," Gary said with resignation in his voice. Vitamins, he knew, were all they could afford.

The African physicians also inquired about linen from patients sick with AIDS and about disposal of the body.

Sitting in the audience with her colleagues, Dr. Leonora Chiposi of Zimbabwe found the discussion interesting. Asked afterward what she did for AIDS patients in her country, she said she could do no more than "sympathy management."

As Gary and Clement walked back to Ward 86, Gary thought that when the epidemic had ended in the United States, he'd go to Africa.

Back at his desk, Gary had to deal with a patient who'd come in with lymphoma, what Gary called "the grand booby prize." The more the nurses and doctors did to prevent Pneumocystis, the more cases of lymphoma they'd see, and it made Gary feel terrible. To no one in particular, he said, "It's not my fault. It's just that it's so sad and it makes me feel powerless."

Gary didn't socialize much with his patients, but Neil, the cat breeder, yoga instructor, rapscallion, had been the exception. For years, he'd come in every Monday morning for medical care and therapeutic schmoozing. Neil was in his late twenties and had lost his health insurance. Away from work, Gary took Neil for a ride to the coastal town of Bolinas on his motorcycle. The two went to the theater together. Then one Monday morning Neil showed up looking awful. One man in his Kaposi's sarcoma support group had slowly choked to death. Neil said he hoped that when it was his turn, he'd go faster than that. Despite chemotherapy and an experimental drug, Neil was failing. One night, Neil and Gary went to a Chinese restaurant where they shared Szechuan prawns, and Gary thought someone who could eat with such gusto couldn't be that sick. Two days later, Neil called. He was having difficulty breathing. Admitted to the General, Neil was given an oxygen mask. Gary offered to stay but Neil sent him away. By morning, Neil was dead. His oxygen mask lay on the bed next to him. It seemed to Gary that, by removing his mask, Neil had committed suicide.

The hardest patients for Gary were the youngest, such as Carlos, who died when he was twenty-two. Born in Cuba, his family had fled to Miami. Carlos had left home at thirteen, making his way to Times Square, back to Miami, and, after someone gave him a one-way bus ticket, to San Francisco, where he lived on the streets, selling himself and using drugs. Carlos had wanted to be a model, but shingles broke out across his forehead. In 1984, he had gone to see Gary about the swollen lymph nodes popping up all over his body. Four years later he was diagnosed with lymphoma and had chemotherapy. His hair thinned until he decided to shave his head. Suddenly, his ears seemed enormous. He didn't want Gary and the other nurses he had known to see him in his debilitated condition. He was moved to Coming Home Hospice, a fifteen-bed facility for dying AIDS patients, tastefully decorated in dusty rose and gray by gay men. On his lunch break or after work, Gary would visit. Toward the end he could see Carlos's ribs. He could practically see his internal organs. He reminded Gary of a concentration camp victim.

"Don't worry about me," he told Gary. "I'll be free. You'll still be trapped in your body." He asked Gary for a message "for the people on the other side." The other side wasn't part of Gary's belief system, but, moved by the patient's sincerity, Gary told him to give a message to the patient with whom he'd fallen in love: "Tell Neil I give him my love and his cat is okay."

Carlos promised and said it was the last time the two would meet, and Gary thought he was right. He told his young friend, "Some day there will be a cure for this disease. When they have a cure, I'll think about you because you're so young."

"Don't worry," Carlos said. "You did your best."

This Little-Old-Lady Bullshit

The old lady didn't see you were out of cookies, guys." One arm was wrapped around a blue-and-white cookie tin, as big as a drum. The other scooped up a few of her 238 (she had counted them) home-baked chocolate-sour-cream-nut cookies, placing them on a plate in the waiting room. Thin men watched TV as she worked. She had been a waitress for fifty-eight years. Now in retirement, the set hair, nylons and bra were gone, but the waitress's cheery demeanor and her convictions remained. Among the pins that traveled down her chest was one reading LEGALIZE MARIJUANA. Beneath it was a large patch with a big green marijuana leaf on a red background. "We're so in need of medical marijuana," she complained. "It must be made available to people on chemotherapy and especially to those with AIDS."

Because of the General's reputation for AIDS care, it has drawn nontraditional volunteers who give the hospital a warmth and character lacking in other institutions.

"Bye bye, honey." She hugged a young man as she slowly headed for the elevators on Ward 86. Every Monday and Thursday afternoon she came. Some called her the cookie lady. Some called her by her real name: Mary Rathbun. Mostly, people just called her Mary, although she also answered to the name Brownie Mary, left over from the days when she sold Alice B. Toklas Brownies to friends and finally, to an undercover cop.

Upon her arrest in 1981, she became a cause célèbre. Her story ran in the London *Times* and in the magazine *High Times* and made front pages in California papers. The police seized thirty-five pounds of margarine, twenty-five pounds of sugar, twenty-five pounds of flour, twenty-two dozen eggs, twenty-one thousand square feet of plastic wrap, twenty-two pounds of high-grade marijuana and fifty-four dozen marijuana brownies. The San Francisco *Examiner* described her arrest succinctly: "Brownie Mary has gone down." At the time she was fifty-seven, doing a brisk business, advertising on telephone poles. She told one of her arresting officers she was smoking dope before he was born. While they searched her home, she sat in her Birkenstocks, pants and Hawaiian shirt, drinking a full glass of bourbon and offering unsolicited advice. When the officers seized trays of cooling pot brownies, she suggested they take them to St. Anthony's Dining Room (which serves free meals to the poor) "and distribute them to the poor souls standing in line." While cordial with reporters, she refused to divulge her recipe, explaining that "old cooks never divulge their recipe, honey." She was waiting until marijuana was legalized "and I sell it to Betty Crocker."

After Mary was ordered to perform five hundred hours of community service, her attorney told the judge about her "terrific spaghetti and dynamite stuffed cabbage," and Mary was allowed to serve her sentence in a soup kitchen. She completed it in two months and "I didn't cheat a bit," she said. "I could have. [The people at the soup kitchen] thought I was the cat's ass."

"Judges don't know jack shit about you," Mary said. To fulfill her sentence, she had to give up her volunteer work at a thrift shop. And when she returned to court, the judge peered over his glasses and said, "I commend you for your total and complete rehabilitation."

A lot of San Franciscans mourned the demise of her business. The city's downtown plan, she was told, would never have been completed without her. Even the mayor's office was buying them, she said. And while police were searching her home, the sister of a police officer and the dean of a local acting school came by to shop.

Half of Mary's customers were gay. And so were half her friends, "because I live in the faggot zip code. Some people can say that. Some people can't. I can. This epidemic came along and so many of my friends were gay, lesbian, bisexual or who cares?" She leaned against a counter, waiting for specimens to carry to the lab. At sixty-six, with one artificial knee and the other one hurting, she was a runner for the ward.

An AIDS patient interrupted her thoughts for a hug. "I've watched a hundred thousand of them deteriorate and die," Mary said.

She spotted her friend Larry in a bed at the end of the **L**-shaped ward. When she walked with someone down the hallway she moved fast enough. When she thought no one was looking, she walked the slow walk of someone in pain. Larry was fifty-one today and not at all happy about spending his birthday in misery at the hospital. He'd been told he should neither eat nor drink. Mary placed three cookies in a plastic sandwich bag for him to take home. He wanted his medication and he wanted to go home. Normally, the patient had to go down to the first-floor pharmacy and wait two hours for a prescription.

"Let's see if I can pull that little-old-lady bullshit and get your pills for you," Mary said.

She scooted out the door and down the hall. While waiting for the elevator she observed, "If I win the lottery, I'm donating an elevator expressly to 86."

"He's sicker than a dog," she said to herself. "I'm not lying."

At the pharmacy window she pleaded with a somber Asian pharmacist. "He's desperately sick. He has no one to wait for him. He's just really sick, honey." To herself, she added, "He's just really sick." The pharmacist accepted her request.

"A half an hour."

"Half an hour is better than two," Mary said. Most of the time, Mary wouldn't have had to plead. "I bribe Sandy [the person usually at the window] with cookies."

She began volunteering at age thirteen, after she had been thrown out of Catholic school for, among other crimes, smoking cigarettes behind the statue of the Virgin Mary. She took the opportunity to run away from home, switching schools and finding a job as a soda jerk. Soon she improved her status, waitressing at "a silver service" restaurant. All might have gone well had an uncle not noticed her there. He told her boss her age, and that got her fired. By the age of twenty, Mary and her girlfriends headed for California.

When AIDS began to spread, Mary volunteered at the Shanti Project in San Francisco, making dinners for her boys, doing their laundry, their banking and mothering them. She made a lot of meatloaf, roast pork, mashed potatoes and gravy. Booze for anyone who asked. That was before the city started funding the Shanti Project and alcohol was outlawed.

Pushing open the heavy glass door, then lighting up a cigarette, Mary headed for the clinical labs in another building and told about her present situation: "Four kids I'm helping who are really sick—Dale, My Tony, Gordy, he's not doing well either . . ." Her voice trailed off. She visited them, cooked for them and, for those who needed it, took them food, when she could afford it.

"How are you doing, sweetie?" she asked a patient, on returning from the lab.

"Fair."

"Fair is better than no good," she said in part because there was nothing she could do for him. Nearby, an earnest-looking chaplain, with eyes full of faith, comforted a patient. Mary's style was decidedly different.

As she took another specimen over to the lab, Mary walked, smoked and cried. "All of us are going to die. Let's face it. We're just born to die.

"Me. I don't give a shit, but these are kids—thirty and thirty-five. Our society teaches life. Don't you dare join the Hemlock Society. That's what our fucking religions teach us. So these boys don't want to die. They've just begun to live."

She bore the sweetness of age and the fury of a witness. "Every once in a while I get so fucking mad at this fucking thing." She cried, while trying to shield herself from the patients she called "my kids." She just talked to a man abandoned by his lover the night before. "Of all the times to leave! I try to be Miss Sunshine. Shit!"

Once, in the main building, she spotted an empty wheelchair and declared it the property of Ward 86. The receptionist with a lilting Irish brogue wasn't about to challenge her. "I used to be known as the wheelchair thief," Mary said with the pride of a righteous burglar. Once, too, she had watched an "old lady my age. She was probably a hypochondriac. She was sitting in the wheelchair," waiting for her X ray. The doctor signaled her to come in. The woman rose from the chair, entered the room and the door was shut. That was when Mary stole the wheelchair and brought it up to Ward 86. She explains, "The patients' mothers buy them for our kids and [the other people in the hospital] steal them!"

She went back to Larry, the birthday man who was still suffering. A nurse said the concern was constipation. "What the hell. Take Metamucil," Mary advised.

She stopped by the book that held name after name of patients from Ward 86 who've died. "It really hurts to see these names. I knew these kids so well.

"They really tried. They all figured they would be the one to make it.

"Ten kids on this page I knew. This one, he was a doctor on 5A. Skip, we used to call him Skippy Peanut Butter."

"Have you ever made beer?" A chair away from Mary, one young doctor talked to another between patients. "I got a starter kit," one said. "It was like drinking ale."

J.B. Molaghan, the nurse with superball bounce, was conferring with a doctor. His smile was gone: "He's going down so fast. I feel awful. He was so handsome. . . . It's awful. Terrible. He's basically just going to die. It's so sad." The patient's family would look after him. He would quickly become a young invalid and then he would die. "I don't want to give up on him," J.B. said.

Some floral thank-you notes appeared in the death book. Others, such as the one from Nebraska Williams's mother, were taped to the door. It read in part: "The word AIDS is so explosive in this area and a gay with AIDS is the lowest dregs of humanity. . . ." She thanked the staff because "you all really cared for him as a person and not as a case." The letter was signed "Just a mom."

In the hallway, Mary hugged Dan Turner, probably the longest-living AIDS patient in San Francisco. The grandmotherly Mary consoled Turner, a remnant of himself. After his diagnosis in 1981, he'd helped start most of the AIDS organizations in the city. Now he was wasting and coughing. He was, he said, "in a crisis situation." He said he was coming back the next day for an appointment with Volberding. Bogged down with administrative tasks, the physician didn't see many AIDS patients any longer, but Dan was one of the few.

Volberding is one of Mary's heroes. "I once saw him crying on the phone. I remember that as clearly as my name is Mary. Doctors, nurses, nurse practitioners. They're the unsung heroes. You can get volunteers. Where are you going to get respected people in the straight community?"

She does not suffer pretentions well. She tucked her arm under Larry's and accompanied him downstairs for his prescription and to a waiting cab. She took another smoke. As she has heroes, so, too, does she have people for whom she reserves "voodoo pins." A lot of them are parents of AIDS patients. As she puffed away, she told the story of her friend James. He was dying with AIDS when his wealthy parents came down from Seattle. They denied that he was gay, claiming he'd contracted the disease in India. They'd come to see him die.

"He lived in the darlingest apartment on Polk Street." Other apartment residents arranged to give the parents an apartment in the building during their stay. Yet when James died, "His mother was out, having her Goddamn fucking hair fixed."

James died surrounded by friends but no family. He had wanted Gary Carr, head nurse practitioner at Ward 86, who kept James as comfortable as possible, to have his ring. For another friend, he had left a picture frame and clock. A lacquered incense box was to go to Mary.

"The parents took everything before James's best friend," to whom he had given power of attorney, "had a chance to say jack shit."

After his death, the father told Mary, "James has come back to the church." Mary and James's other friends sought their revenge. She chuckled as she recalled it. The Names quilt was on its way to Seattle with James's panel on it.

She stamped out her cigarette, popped the butt in her pocket and headed back to work with her "kids."

Common Sense

I don't want to be a hypochondriac but I've just been having weird stuff." His small face twitched. Legs and arms were in flight. He'd come for his daily dose of methadone and for his AIDS examination. Stories spilled out of him. He's HIV positive. His wife is, too, and she's becoming sick. Today is his daughter's birthday and "It's fucked." He thought the disease might be "exacerbating my nervousness." Lately, he said, he'd been trembling "like a marionette." (He's full of what another ex-addict called "twenty-five cent words.")

Dr. Eric Goosby asked if the patient had been emotionally upset. The patient said he hadn't been. He complained of light-headedness, ringing in his ears, pain in his arms. His said he couldn't wait until nine each night when he could sleep.

With earnest eyes, the patient focused on the physician and moved onto other symptoms. He had a pain in his chest and a knot in his stomach, pain in his legs that made him think he was an old man. "I need something for my fucking nerves. Phenobarbital? May as well give me sugar pills. I sleep all right at night. It's getting through the day without being freaked. Have you got something that can calm me down a little bit?"

Goosby limited his prescription to phenobarbital anyway. "What's your number?" he asked.

"My hospital card number or my prison number?" the patient replied.

Goosby was still learning about IV drug users. Educated in the traditional medical model, he wanted to believe his patients were telling him the truth. Not to believe them made him feel uncomfortable. From a prominent black San Francisco family, he'd grown up with a sense of civic obligation. (His father had been the president of the San Francisco School Board.) He began his career as an AIDS doctor working with gays. IV drug users were something else.

Over and over again, patients did whatever they could to get sleep medicines, pain medicines or more methadone. The internist was constantly being "barraged by these very talented people." They were tricking him "left and right."

Dealing with AIDS was an education of the emotions. By the summer of 1989, it wasn't at all clear how much longer Goosby could tolerate his patients' daily campaign of misinformation.

He knew that the patient he was examining wanted Valium, although the patient never asked for it by name. Valium would give him a better buzz than phenobarbital. More and more Goosby had been working with patients who'd contracted the disease from shared needles. Many of them lived under freeway overpasses, in hallways and up against downtown buildings—with regular sojourns in jail. They rose when the sun went down. Some stole for a living. Industrious ones picked through dumpsters in search of things to sell.

Patients with scruffy hair, missing teeth, bad eyes, limps, canes and crutches walked around the old red-brick Building 80, which housed Ward 86 to the side entrance of Building 90. They punched the elevator button for the methadone clinic. On the wall above the receptionist the sign read NO DEALING. NO WEAPONS. NO VIOLENCE. NO THREATS.

In the sparse hallway, the men and women hugged, touched and chatted while waiting for their daily dose of methadone. On this particular day they talked about one of their own who recently drove a new car that wasn't hers and got caught. She was returned to jail. A client dropped off three boxes of sour suckers. Next to the lollipops a plastic kidney dish was filled with silver packets of Life Style condoms. The stock of lollipops immediately dwindled. Nobody touched the condoms.

Methadone clinics had to be run with almost militaristic regulation. If a client failed to show up he was given a warning. After repeated offenses, he could be thrown out of the program. Twice a month, spot drug checks were conducted. If a person was found to be positive for heroin, cocaine, Tylenol-Codeine, Valium or other drugs, he was advised to enter a rehab program. If he was caught again, he was pushed out of the program.

AIDS had altered the rules. An HIV-positive patient was never thrown out of the methadone program. Dr. Steven Batki, a psychiatrist and medical director of substance abuse services at the General, bent the rules for infected drug users because whenever HIV-positive patients quit taking their methadone, they were more likely to return to the streets, share needles and transmit the virus.

Nearly everyone at the methadone clinic at the General could have been a drab extra at the big city bus terminal. Jennifer was an exception, with sparkling orange rhinestoned nails so long they curved like claws. Her dyed red hair and her strong personality made her the leading lady of the hallway. She shouted to friends and doctors, offering advice.

"I need to speak to you," said the down-to-earth Goosby in a somber tone. His usual smile was gone.

She followed him into a small exam room. "The pharmacy has talked to me about the prescription I wrote for you," he said.

She pretended not to know what was coming next.

On each prescription pad five spaces were demarcated for prescriptions. Goosby had prescribed the nutritional supplement Ensure and drawn lines through the other four spaces. Jennifer probably had spent an hour or two artfully erasing and rewriting the prescription to give herself Klonopin, an antianxiety drug ten times more powerful than Valium. Having seen patients with artistic talent before, the hospital pharmacy had not been conned.

Jennifer was full of bravado. "I asked you to write me a letter before you went on vacation. I never got it. I had a lot of legal problems with my parole officer and the judge. Because I couldn't get the letter I got stressed out. [Goosby had written the letter. She hadn't picked it up.] I needed the Klonopin. I figured you owed it to me."

Goosby was used to treating gay AIDS patients with values much like his own. Many were his age. As an internist, he'd grown accustomed to patients dying. But he'd never grieved the way he grieved for some of his AIDS patients. And when they died, he felt the awful emptiness and insanity of it all. Lately he'd been seeing the third wave, gay men who had been the support system for those who had died before. Now, when some of them visited their favorite gay bars they could find no one left they knew. Families had abandoned them. The physician sometimes became their main human contact. AIDS, Goosby felt, compressed the distance between patient and physician. While he was seeing Jennifer he was treating a gay (non-drug-using) AIDS patient whose doctors in Louisiana had isolated him at the local hospital and suggested that if he wanted good care he should go to San Francisco. The patient's well-to-do mother bought him a one-way airline ticket and gave him money to set himself up in the new city. He was twenty-one. Goosby had great empathy for the young man.

He also had great empathy for many of the IV-drug-using AIDS patients. Most of them had led horrible lives. But when he dealt with patients like Jennifer, he felt manipulated. He was used to seeing patients cry when they were dying, not when he refused to prescribe Valium or Klonopin.

"This makes me not trust you," he told Jennifer. "I consider it a transgression. It's illegal and I'm personally offended. If anything like this happens in the future, I'm not going to be able to take care of you. We'll have to get you another doctor."

For fifteen years, Jennifer had been abused by her mother's boyfriend. At sixteen, she had run away to San Francisco, where she had worked for a pimp. Even while on methadone and being treated for AIDS, she remained a prostitute except for the times she spent in jail. It made the physician wonder whether, if he had gone through what she had, he could have survived.

Jennifer left the exam room with her bravado intact and immediately caught up with her friend Crystal. They made an odd pair. Jennifer was still kidlike, white and full of herself; age forty but looking sixty-five, Crystal was older, black and defeated. Doodling was the only thing she enjoyed in life. She kept her bus pass, pencil and paper in a jeans-colored briefcase. On the briefcase, Jennifer had affixed a pin for her friend. It said LIVE YOUR DREAMS.

At 102 pounds, down from 150, Crystal had thick cheeks, an overhanging forehead and a body that was needle thin. She hadn't been able to eat in several days. For years she'd survived on the streets trading in anything "stealable." With eclectic tastes, she stole silk dresses, tools, checks out of the mail and what she simply called "Apples." The computers, she said, weren't hot. "They didn't even have serial numbers on them yet." As she spoke, a nurse came by to beg her to drink a cup of water.

"The grass aint hasn't been green," Crystal said. She was hoping not to live too much longer. "If you see a little kid who needs kidneys they can take these 'cause I'm real tired. Nothing else here for me. I'm not contributing. I'm sick with this virus." (It didn't occur to her that because she was carrying the virus, her organs could not be transplanted into anyone.)

Several of Goosby's IV-drug-using AIDS patients roamed the hallway. Whatever corridors Tiffany traveled, trouble ensued. Typically she screamed, cried and threw tantrums at the front desk, when she stopped by without an appointment. Recently, when the wait was too long, she let loose, calling AIDS nurses "faggot fuckers." Security guards hauled her away. That proved, she said, how little compassion the staff had for her.

"The way they treat you is the shits. You don't feel good. You're afraid. Nobody wants to see you. My body hurts. Just write me a prescription. . . . I'm tired of being put down and made to feel worse," Tiffany said while waiting for a doctor. "They take my dignity and squash it."

The methadone clients seemed to like Tiffany. To the hospital staff she was a disruptive influence.

She rose from her waiting-room seat and headed for the nursing station, where she demanded to see someone. Tiffany had minimal ARC, the precursor to AIDS. Her physical ailments were minor compared with those of the majority of wasted men waiting to see a nurse or doctor. She spoke freely about how she missed being close to her mother. But whenever Tiffany visited, her mother insisted she wear gloves.

Because of her noisy presence, Tiffany rarely had to wait very long to see someone. The staff was always anxious for her to leave. "People have tried to meet her halfway," Goosby said. "She never approached it."

With many of the other ex-addicts, Goosby had a far better rapport.

His patient James had been battling the hospital system for several years before they met. James still wore the leather and pointed metal "violence bracelet" designed to puncture a face in a fight, but his husky, weightlifter body had been cut to a sliver. In his heyday, he'd committed armed robberies, passed bad checks and been involved in credit-card fraud. He had spent two years in college and two years in prison.

Not long ago, when he had been hospitalized, he threatened a doctor who refused to give him his full dose of methadone. "If you don't give me the seventy milligrams I'll report you and I'll have your ass, not just your job," James had said. "If you go home at night, I'll wait for you and break your arm."

When nurses on Ward 86 had asked James if he wanted to participate in an experimental drug study, he became infuriated, calling them "dirt bags." He thought they were saying "Your life isn't worth two cents." Goosby understood that James interpreted the study as research on "dead meat." "It wasn't a bad thing," the physician said. "It was a miscommunication."

James felt he was part of a two-tiered system: the gays (or the haves) and the drug users (the have-nots.) He surveyed the waiting area of the AIDS outpatient unit and felt he had "nothing in common with these people, except the virus."

His medical folder at the General was thick. For his appointments, James arrived with his own medical file, tucked into a Black Jack cigar box. One day, after James had been tossed from one physician to the next, Goosby approached him. "Would you consider working with me?" the physician asked, and it made James go weak in the knees. James showed respect for his doctor because he felt the respect in return. "I'd rather cut my finger off than tell him an untruth," James said. He felt Goosby cared for him more than his family had. "They dropped me like I was a bad habit."

Sometimes the backdoor message from the doctors to IV drug users and ex-users is "you're something less than human," Goosby said. He tries not to judge those patients. He doesn't need to tell them that shooting up is bad for them. So he moves on from there and treats them medically.

"We don't need to make a moral judgment," Goosby said. "That's the wonderful thing about being a doctor. We're not priests. We may feel their behavior increases the [health] risks. It's our job to make sure they understand the risks. It's not our job to tell them they're bad and doing something wrong."

In time, Goosby adjusted to the lies and manipulation. He came to appreciate ex-addicts' smarts and strength. He quit taking any single incident too seriously, preferring to see what he called the gestalt of a patient. And when he treated them as equals, they responded. "I can count on one hand the number of people on whom it hasn't worked," he said. Tiffany was one. In the fall of 1990, after doing jail time for prostitution, she returned to the streets, shot up heroin and died of an overdose, not of AIDS.

James was still alive. As his T cells dropped, his will to live rose. He began seeing his grown daughter again and formed a relationship with one of the other methadone clients.

Goosby found the hardened drug-using patients appreciative. They didn't bring flowers or gifts. But when the physician had left his wallet in the clinic and had no cash to buy a sandwich at the canteen truck at lunchtime, four or five of his patients standing in line took up a collection.

Goosby and the other physicians and nurses were doling out more than medical care to the members of what he called "this lost group."

"They liked to be taken seriously and have their needs met in a way that shows you respect them. That's not a magical formula," Goosby said. "It's just common sense."

"Those who had never felt human warmth just took a little longer to respond. There are certain universal things," he said. "This is one."

Motel Room 117

"In the last six months, how many male partners have you had?"

"Shiiiiit!"

"Okay. On an average. How many tricks in a week?"

"That's hard to say."

"In a day?"

"Seven to ten."

"Were any of these men bisexual or gay?"

"Not to my knowledge."

"Any IV drug users?"

"Not that I know of. If they're a date, I just use rubbers. I don't worry."

"How about with your man?"

"No. I tried to slip one on him with my tongue. He didn't think it was funny at all."

Georgette was smoking, yawning, impatient, tweaking, coming off the peak of a cocaine high. She was on, but sliding. She walked and talked in hyperspeed: "Iwanttogetbacktoworkwhen'sthisgoingtobeover?"

A black jersey stopped short at her ample midriff; black Spandex with a turquoise streak hugged her thighs. She packed 150 dollars from her morning's work in her electric-blue spike heels. In the folds of her sleeves and tucked into her waist she has jammed more condoms than one person is allowed at this, the Association for Women's AIDS Research and Education (AWARE) outing. She was like the kid at Halloween who's offered one Reese's Peanut Butter Cup but when a back is turned grabs five more.

She knew nothing about Dr. Day, Jane Doe, Q trials or the hospital setting. In exchange for some food, camaraderie, cash, AIDS-test results and condoms, she was willing to help the researchers learn about the transmission of the AIDS virus among women.

"Please be patient," said a husky female "dope fiend in recovery" named Black Star. An ill-suited couple, Black Star sat in the driver's seat marking down answers on a questionnaire, while Georgette fidgeted in the passenger's seat of the parked Hyundai. In numerous parking spaces, in nondescript compact cars, interviewers questioned the prostitutes. To a passerby, the lot with the parked vehicles and clipboard interviews resembled the department of motor vehicles before a driver's test.

Twice a month, the crowd from San Francisco General and UCSF drives to Oakland's seedy MacArthur Boulevard, where prostitutes have paraded for decades. Epidemiologists, doctors, nurses and outreach workers set up shop on a block cluttered with hotels but no tourists. They use two motel rooms and half the parking lot with their cars and one long, tan van in which blood is drawn and exams are provided. Down the block the Lucky Florist shop abuts a mortuary. Men without work take their time walking the block. Young women in tight clothes wave and shout at passing motorists. Here at the Travel Inn—DIAL PHONES AND COLOR TV—epidemiologiust Dr. Judith Cohen meets up with her subjects.

A big, lively woman, Cohen has a slightly disheveled look that would probably disqualify her from a corporate post or a bank job, which she couldn't stand anyway. In the forefront of research on women and AIDS, her interest developed simply, logically. She'd been working on a routine epidemiological AIDS study when, back in 1984, a small group of women hanging around the coffee machine agreed, "There's no reason why women aren't going to get this disease."

"Nobody would take us seriously because everyone up there [doing the research] was a man. Yet we knew from other sexually transmitted diseases it was going to happen," Cohen said. By 1985, only three women in San Francisco had been diagnosed with AIDS. Two of them had acquired the virus from blood transfusions and the third was believed to have gotten it from a male sex partner. Dr. Constance Wofsy, one of the early AIDS doctors and one of the women at the coffee machine, saw several of the other early women. "They were drugs users," said Cohen, "So they were kind of not [average] women because they were drug users." The Centers for Disease Control had not even created a category for heterosexual transmission. "Common sense," Cohen said, "was not a part of the picture yet."

One august medical journal published a letter saying women couldn't get AIDS because various labs had been unable to grow the AIDS virus from vaginal secretions. AWARE asked women to donate vaginal and cervical secretions. From the samples, Dr. Jay Levy, one of the first scientists to isolate the AIDS virus, grew the virus. His findings were published in *Lancet* in 1986.

"We were getting calls from women who were going to their doctors and their doctors were saying, 'Don't worry. Women can't get it.' We couldn't get any interest to look at it in a research sense," Cohen recalled.

All that changed on January 5, 1985, when one single, dramatic news story appeared in the *San Francisco Chronicle*. Reporter Randy Shilts told of a prostitute with AIDS who was taken to the General by police escort and released. "I don't like the idea of maybe giving this to someone else, but I don't have any other way to survive other than to work the street," said the unnamed prostitute, in one sentence doing more to shut down the streetwalker trade than an entire police vice squad could have. In the article, Volberding called the issue "a monster," pitting public health against the woman's civil rights. Also interviewed for the article, Wofsy said the woman needed AIDS services when none were available for women in general and prostitutes in particular.

The story had unanticipated effects. A crowd of suburban husbands with guilty consciences showed up at the old red-brick building that housed Ward 86, the outpatient unit, convinced they had the symptoms. For a few days, nurses on the ward spent more time being shrinks than administering medical care.

For Cohen, the article's effects were more beneficial: "All of a sudden everybody was worried about women and AIDS." The Mayor's Task Force on AIDS called its first meeting on heterosexual transmission. A number of women, Cohen included, offered to attend the gathering instead of their male bosses. Some of the top physicians remained skeptical. "We probably ought to look into it," Cohen remembered one saying, "but there's probably no way to study it."

"Everyone agreed it was laudatory to study women," the epidemiologist said. "But they wouldn't necessarily fund it. They were interested in our studying prostitutes because that's what they were worried about."

Wofsy, Cohen and associates received forty thousand dollars from the state of California for a four-month study. The money, Cohen was sure, was supposed to be a cheap way of proving the women wrong. "I'm sure they were thinking it really wasn't feasible. That we wouldn't find anything. That no one would cooperate. That it was a nonissue."

Four or five young women lounge on each of two beds with mismatched floral spreads, chattering like college girls after a big weekend. The décor is mustard drab. The carpets are pocked with holes. Windows are protected by black metal bars. The women are grabbing free condoms. "I don't know why they're taking them," Georgette says. In joking, haughty tones she adds, "I work the most." Her dark skin is offset by her bleached golden hair in tiny rope braids and Grecian-style ponytail with a silverish conical clasp. Through the rouge and Cleopatra eye pencil appears a round, intelligent face.

No matter how many condoms they're given, they want more. In 1985, when AWARE began, only 18 percent of the working women were insisting their men wear condoms. Four years later, the figure had risen to 78 percent. "Even with your man it's unsafe," Georgette advised. "You don't know who he slept with way back when." Although Georgette is knowledgeable, her life insurance policy doesn't extend to boyfriends.

"Get your veins ready," a friend joked.

"They want your pelvic veins," Georgette said with a laugh.

Cohen distributes "The Hot and Sexy Safe Sex Contest: Grand Prize $100; Second Prize 100 Condoms." Sponsored by various AIDS and prostitution groups, it's a multiple-choice contest. For each sex or drug act described, the respondent is to mark the answer: "safe," "possibly safe" or "unsafe." The twenty questions include "Getting a blow job without a condom," "Cunnilingus/going down on a woman," "Body-to-body rubbing," "Fisting without a latex glove," "Cleaning IV needles with bleach," "Hand job/jacking off" and other graphic sex acts. The women giggle. "A hand job is safe unless you got a cut on your hand," Georgette said, her elbow shoved against a pillow.

As they talk, a former prostitute turned outreach worker and professional educator spreads mayo on white bread, making sandwiches for the women.

Despite the research being conducted and the seriousness of the subject, the prostitutes camouflage their concern in laughter. And the outreach workers blend in. As she collected the Hot and Sexy Safe Sex Contest quiz, Cohen observed: "Life doesn't have to be negative even when it seems to be going out of its way to be."

Initially the federal government's interest in women and AIDS was limited to testing the blood of prostitutes. The CDC sent out a request for proposal for a "survey of HIV infection among prostitutes." The survey had no provisions for confidentiality, counseling or notification. Women were to be interviewed in jails and drug treatment programs, or what Cohen characterized as coercive settings.

Calling the plan unethical, Cohen warned the CDC that its findings were likely to be inaccurate and that its plan was just plain wrong. Then she told them how they ought to do it and what questions needed to be asked. "Needless to say, we captured their attention." In a surprising turnaround for the federal bureaucracy, the CDC agreed to Cohen's plan.

San Francisco's success was persuasive. At the first meeting, collaborators from other cities reported that they had found three, five or seven prostitutes for testing. San Francisco General had 120. Other collaborators had blood but no information. "When you have a jail staff asking behavioral questions, do you really think the women will give honest and complete answers?" Cohen said with a chortle. In Florida, researchers rode around in police cars, handing out cards asking the women to come in and be part of their study. "Then they couldn't understand why nobody showed up." Desperate to find women, New Jersey investigators made participation a condition of women's enrollment in a methadone program. "Guess how many drug users they had in their study?" Cohen said. The New Jersey infection rate was phenomenally higher than that anywhere else. But their findings were based not on prostitutes but on drug users. "Those," said Cohen, "were fine points."

It was about then that Cohen began seeing things the way activist prostitutes did. "I started out being this scientist and more and more I kept getting hot under the collar at these blindnesses that took my breath away. It was not just prejudice. It was," she said, "a lack of common sense."

Like a lot of other people working on AIDS at the General, she had come of age in the '60s. Radicalized, she believed that she could be both objective and humane. Her commitment to helping prostitutes, drug users and other stigmatized women grew. "My whole experience has made me more active and more service oriented than I'm supposed to be as an epidemiologist," she said. "I don't get points for this with the university. One reason this program works is that it's not pure research. It's a creative, chaotic blend of epidemiology and advocacy and a funny, eclectic mix of people."

Her program failed to fit into a neat medical model. Instead of top down, it was from the bottom up. Cohen and associates consulted their would-be subjects. They sought advice from prostitutes'-rights groups, women's conferences, feminist groups and health-care providers. Prostitutes told the researchers that if they were going to be interviewed it had better be by people who spoke their language and not by bureaucrats using too much medical terminology. And if they participated, the prostitutes said, they also wanted advice and referrals when needed.

Cohen understood their other needs as well. Terrified women had been calling the General. They wanted to know if they were going to die of AIDS, but they didn't want to give their names or telephone numbers and they didn't want to go to AIDS clinics.

Wofsy and Cohen set up a series of conditions for studying the women at risk for AIDS. They would not be required to come to an AIDS clinic. They would not have to give their name, social security number or telephone number. And they could talk to people much like themselves. Finding such staff was easy compared to putting them on the University of California Medical School payroll. The school maintained its own list of qualified interviewers, but Cohen wasn't buying. "I can't take uptight, university educated interviewers and make them comfortable on the streets." Someone dressed for success "would get laughed off the street or mugged." Filling out job applications wasn't so simple. What was a woman supposed to say about her background? Searching for an appropriate euphemism to placate personnel, Cohen came up with "counseling around sexual dysfunction" and "health educator." The former prostitutes and drug users were hired.

"Are you pregnant?"

"No," Georgette says with a laugh. "I had my tubes tied. I done should had them tied years ago." At twenty-nine, she has five kids. Three of them live with her. "What's your zip code?"

"I don't know."

She's given a code number to retrieve the results of her AIDS test. "Do you think you could get AIDS?"

"Yeah. Anybody can." The two discuss how to contract the disease. Georgette is well informed.

"Sometimes I might laugh a little bit. But this is serious stuff. I'm sometimes embarrassed," Black Star says. She asks Georgette about her sexual activity since 1980. "Are you straight-up men or do you do women?"

"Straight-up men," Georgette replies, looking askance.

Black Star continues, quizzing Georgette about the number of sexual partners she's had with the fluidity of someone surveying TV habits.

"Precious Lord . . . Lead me on . . . I am tired . . ." In the parking lot, the surreal sounds of melodic gospel flow. The prostitute looks thin, tired. Her singing uplifts her and everybody around. On her button-down shirt she wears a pin that ill suits the song: ORGASM FOR SALE RENT OR TRADE.

On the street a blond prostitute in remarkably clinging white dress and pink high heels mosies by. She's model pretty, until she smiles, exhibiting a large gap between her front teeth. She laughs in a carefree way. Her manner deceives. She'd already taken a blood test and learned she is HIV positive. Now, she's back.

Pamela, an outreach worker and former prostitute who earned four hundred to six hundred dollars a night in hotels, had been the one to give her the results. When the results came in, outreach workers took to the streets, looking for the women. Those who were pregnant were given their results sooner. Infected women have a one-in-three chance of passing the disease on to their infants. Nevertheless, UCSF researchers have found that invariably such women choose to continue their pregnancies.

Telling someone she carries the virus is the hardest part of Pamela's job. It makes her feel she's giving a woman "a death sentence." The outreach worker tries to be strong, although sometimes she can't help but cry, too. Usually a woman wants to know if she's going to die. And if she's a mother, she asks, "Who will care for my children?" Pamela thinks the disease "is about one-hundred percent fatal," but she can't bear to steal someone's hope, so she says, "It does not necessarily mean you're going to die." She tells them it's a serious disease.

Pamela talks about condoms, about not breastfeeding, about services that are available. She holds the woman's hand, wipes away tears or takes the woman's face in her hands. "I want to let them know it's not horrible. It's okay for me to touch them even though I know they're infected. They're afraid no one will want to touch them or love them again."

Pamela spots the lady in white and gives her a hug. The HIV-positive woman is back on the streets. After receiving her results, she'd quit street work remaining with her steady boyfriend. But when he was in an accident, becoming paralyzed and confined to a wheelchair, she returned to making money the only way she knew. "We come from a nonjudgmental area," Pamela said. "We don't say, 'You know you shouldn't work.' We say, 'You should always use condoms.'" HIV-positive women are given more condoms than those who are negative.

"Tongue kissing?"

"I don't."

"With your old man?"

"He's not that affectionate. He's very mean."

"Is that your pimp?"

"If that's what you want to call him."

"Does he go down on you?"

"Yeah."

"Do your dates?"

"Yeah."

"Do you go down on your dates?"

"I do have a lot of oral-cop dates because a lot of guys in Oakland don't have the money to screw."

"Do these people come in your mouth?"

"Oh, no! How can you do that with a rubber?" Georgette religiously uses condoms. Except for the times when she doesn't.

She interrupts the interview for a check of Black Star's credentials. "You never worked the streets before?"

"I shot dope," Black Star explained, turning back to her list of questions: "Do you straight-up fuck?"

"Sometimes. Most don't have the money to screw me."

"Do you have sex on your period?"

"I put a sponge on. I can't stop working 'cause I'm going to bleed for a week."

"Do you butt fuck?"

"I don't do that with anyone."

She's asked about sex toys. "I used to work with Big Al. I used to perform with dildos. They were mine."

Asked about her current risk for AIDS, Georgette says, "I always use condoms."

"Do you refuse men who don't wear them?"

"Yeah."

"Your man doesn't let you wear a condom with him, right?"

"Yeah."

Black Star asks about "Steady partners. Like people who are close to your heart." Georgette says she's had three in the last six months.

"Since 1980?"

"Oh, gosh. I don't know."

She talks about Richie, Bobby and Charles. They've probably never been tested for AIDS, she said. One is from Haiti. Another has spent time in prison. All have multiple partners. She says she slept with Charles about every other day. With five women, "It was like you take turns. You work your way up to his bedroom. Why not leave all this out?"

"Please be patient, okay? After this you get your blood test and your money."

For her participation, Georgette would receive ten dollars.

"I know it's like bullshit. Just be patient."

The explicit questions that sometimes irritated Georgette were needed, Cohen explained, to study the relative risk of AIDS transmission. "If we're going to have safe-sex advice that's current and gives people options, we need this information." Her study would dispel myths, such as the one that women could only contract the AIDS virus through anal sex. In fact, what her study found was that the women most likely to be HIV positive were those who were intravenous drug users. The second most likely group of women to have the virus were those with steady partners who were IV drug users. The third group were those whose steady male partners had sex with other men.

Relieved that the interview was over, Georgette waited to have her blood drawn. Whiling away the time, she tried to trade one cigarette for a handful of condoms. "That's crazy!" a nurse declared. "Cigarettes kill you. Condoms save you." When she finished her cigarettes, Georgette used her Salem cigarette box as a condom holder.

"You going to take me back to work?" she asked Black Star as she tumbled out of the car.

"Say what?"

Georgette walked over to the huge tan trailer that served as a mobile medical clinic for prostitutes. With peach-colored curtains and a kitchen table, it looked like a vacation home that might be parked at Niagara Falls for Mom, Dad and the kids. Inside were two nurses, Dr. Wofsy and three women having their blood drawn.

Georgette waited impatiently. She was anxious to return to work. "I might stop at three hundred dollars. I might come back out tonight." Moments later, she was negotiating with an outreach worker for more condoms. "A lot of girls will be lying. They say they use condoms and they don't," she said. Inside the van, a nurse was searching for a vein on a drug-using prostitute. Georgette claimed she could find one: "Let me go to the back of her legs."

The gospel singer halted her serenade: "She ain't got no veins."

"So what did you used to do?" Georgette asked outreach worker Pamela.

"I used to work."

"Where?"

"Hollywood," Pamela said and smiled.

The door to the van opened. Georgette entered. As her blood was being taken, she asked, "Did you used to work the streets?"

"Never did," the nurse said easily.

"Oh, you're a nurse."

In the front part of the van, the doctor was questioning a plump prostitute named Nicole, who wore a black bodysuit. Her hand protected with a glove, Wofsy drew blood.

In a motel room, epidemiologist Cohen received the blood and prepared it to be sent by overnight delivery to the Centers for Disease Control and to a local lab for testing.

An early afternoon humor had evolved into warmth and joviality in motel room 117. A nineteen-year-old who joked that she was a "sexretary," drank a Coke and complained, "They expect you to suck penis without a condom. I tell them, 'No condom. No service.' 'Cause you can die young. It hits you once and you're gone."

As she talked, a three-year-old named Ashley whose hair was decorated with red, yellow and blue barrettes, was having her nails painted by her mother, a young prostitute. "My beautiful baby," the mother said, moving to the next little finger.

By late afternoon, the crowds were gone. "Walk where He leads you. Walk where He leads you," the gospel singer stayed at the motel until the AWARE nurses, doctor and researcher were ready to leave.

"I keep telling her she needs to do something with that voice," another waiting woman said.

An outreach worker cleared Room 117 of the coldcuts lunch. The gospel singer turned to leave. "I really enjoyed myself. You all are real good people."

After her blood was drawn, Georgette socialized for a while with other women and with a few men sitting on the motel steps. Before she left she announced, "I want some more rubbers."

From the Castro

Sure. They knew each other. From the Jacuzzi and the free weights.
Both Harold and Teddy were from the Castro, the center of San
Francisco's gay society, and both worked out at Muscle Systems. They'd
never spoken, yet they'd covered the same ground at the same time.

Before fitness was in fashion, the best disco in town was Trocadero
Transfer. Their awareness of one another, or at least Harold's awareness of the younger, livelier Teddy, went back to the good old days,
when going to Trocadero was like slipping into Shangri-la. "If you were
on the right drugs, had the right music and the right men, it was a
whole other experience in life," said Teddy, sitting on the edge of his
hospital bed, legs kicking the side for emphasis.

At thirty-four, Harold looked like a tanned camp counselor taking a
break from braiding lanyards and reading ghost stories to the kids. He
was a musicologist without a job. Teddy, twenty-nine, claimed he'd
grown up, but that was a euphemism for being on the runway to
adulthood. He resembled a bouncy camper enthusing over volleyball.

They'd come to the General to participate in the GLQ223 (Q) tests. Thousands of patients had wanted McGrath's Q, but these men were some of the chosen. In this, the first stage of the drug trial, Q was being tested for toxicity.

The men were assigned room 332, just down the hall and around the corner from McGrath's lab. Each man was being given an infusion of Q four times over four weeks, and kept for observation each time for twenty-four hours. Q no longer sat in vials on McGrath's lab counter. His in vitro results were being tested in vivo by Teddy and Harold and others.

Both had arrived in jogging pants and T-shirts, the picture of health, which in reality, they weren't. Teddy had slept just fine the night before—after taking two sleeping pills. An insomniac, the prospect of going on Q had made him too excited. Although "it was not the same as going to Great America on the rides," he added.

A clear bag marked GLQ223 hung from the metal tree. The drug dripped through a tube into their arms. Harold and Teddy knew Q was a toxin; they hoped it was a cure. Failing that, they hoped it would buy them time. Every few minutes, nurses came by to draw blood, which was taken to McGrath's lab to be measured for Q levels. Teddy and Harold were guinea pigs, but you couldn't tell from their conversation.

Moments after they'd met, their talk centered neither on their disease nor the risks they were taking that morning, but on sex, which had gotten them into Room 332 in the first place. Both were dating men they called "blondes." Harold said he couldn't be happier, now that he had a satisfying relationship. The effervescent Teddy, with a string of boy-friends over the years, allowed that he was happy, too. As Q dripped into their veins, plumage was flying around the small hospital room. Harold kiddingly suggested that when the blondes came for a visit, he and Teddy might want to "play switcheroos."

They received 240 ccs of GLQ223 over a two-hour period. Pharma-cokinetics—the study of the body's absorption and excretion of drugs—would determine how much was needed to replicate what happened in a petri dish. They began by being infused with the challenge dose of pure Q to be sure they weren't allergic. The rest of the time the infusion was mixed with sugar water.

Teddy compared Trocadero with a defunct New York gay hangout. A star machine had lit up the dance floor. The place was so big that "if you lost your friend, it could take you an hour to find him." People in New

York danced all right, although Teddy said the dancing seemed more intense than it really was, thanks to drugs. He hopped off his bed and did a five-second performance, purely to illustrate.

Dancing at Trocadero was something else again, Harold was saying. "We're talking virtuoso dancing." Their conversation was reminiscent of many in California, a comparison of East and West. They'd arrived at their decisions about Q long before, having spent hours talking to the formal but caring Vince DeGenova, the nurse who selected subjects for the General and UCSF's AIDS drug studies.

The first thing Teddy had asked DeGenova about was the risk of becoming comatose. He knew about the patients at Project Inform, brought out of their comas within a few days with Decadron. He'd heard someone had died. And he knew about Charlie Weaver, the General patient who'd gone into a coma and remained there for nearly two weeks before he was given steroids and only partially recovered.

DeGenova had wanted them to understand that things could happen to a patient on Q, things that were beyond unpleasant. More of the intellectual, Harold had read the accounts in the gay papers. A video-era adult, Teddy relied on a friend "who reads everything" to tell him about Q. Both men had had physicals, EKGs, brain scans to help screen out HIV patients with dementia.

"Basically," said Harold, a blue thermal blanket covering him, "you're taking a chance." Three people at San Francisco General had had exactly the same dosage and one had gone into a coma. "Two people were okay. One was bad. The odds aren't bad."

AIDS alters perspectives. Two doomed young men sat in a small, nearly colorless hospital room talking about how lucky they were. Nurses quietly came and went, drawing blood and taking urine specimens. "I'm a walking talking miracle, and that's not hyperbole," Harold said.

"What's hyperbole?" Teddy asked.

Harold had had a non-Hodgkin's lymphoma that was treated with chemotherapy. He'd lost his hair and, temporarily, his vanity, and the chemo had made him very ill. Nine months later, he was still free "from this aggressive cancer, and that's pretty good."

He was back to tending to his appearance. His hair had grown in. "I feel damn proud of how I look. I know I'm in good shape. I know I look good. I'm a statement about what people can do when you're given the diagnosis of AIDS."

Before Harold learned about his condition he was timid. Once diagnosed, he put his life in order and decided that if he was going to get what he needed he'd have to snap out of his shyness. "It's the most positive change in my life. . . . I'm damned aggressive. . . . I've finally handled my sex life. I've begun to write music again regularly. I'm clear what I want to do." What he wanted to do included working toward a Ph.D. in musicology if and when he was able to beat the disease. Sometimes Harold talked that way and sometimes he didn't. Denial and reality took their turns. "I don't know how long I have to live. I don't want to live the last year or couple of years of my life without having things I want to get."

A black kid with a cap and a smile popped into the room, selling chocolate almond bars, a reminder that not everyone was wrapped up in AIDS.

The two patients continued their stories. A friend of Teddy's, a wealthy property owner, became ill, sold some of his investments and began living off the proceeds. Teddy said his friend joked, "What's going to happen if they come up with a cure? I'll have to go to work again."

Throughout the day, Teddy received telephone calls. He said he had loads of friends. Yet he had taken a taxi unaccompanied to the hospital the morning of his Q infusion. He had contact with his parents back in New Jersey, but he hadn't told them about Q. Harold's parents were dead. His sister knew about the drug test. His twin brother didn't. What intimacy Harold and Teddy had was with their current lovers, "the blondes."

Two hours after the infusion had begun, a buzzer went off on Harold's machine. A nurse disconnected his line. Seven minutes later, Teddy's machine beeped. Neither man felt any different, which was not unusual. If they were going to experience flulike symptoms, the sickness would manifest itself some hours later. Harold and Teddy said they weren't going to get the flu.

Harold had brought several novels and the latest issue of Project Inform's newsletter to read—all about Q. Calling its own data "only suggestive and inconclusive," the researchers wrote that Q appeared to benefit many types of patients after just three infusions. However, it added, "all benefits noted thus far seem temporary, with declines beginning to show up six to eight weeks after treatment. The presence of additional benefits from repeated, regular use, such as once a month, or once per quarter, awaits further study."

Harold might have brought a videotape to watch in the lounge, but he only owns one: *Cinderella.* "I never got over when her dress got poofed."

Teddy came better prepared. He brought *Baghdad Café, Who Framed Roger Rabbit* and *Aria.* They would watch all three.

Teddy knew "exactly when he turned seropositive." Although exactly whom he got the virus from was unknown. In 1983, when Teddy was in the thick of the party scene, he got the febrile illness that often follows exposure and from then on, he'd had chronic lymphadenopathy, a swelling of the lymph nodes that is symptomatic of the AIDS virus. His body had clicked onto red alert. His brain swiveled into denial. "I was still partying, dancing, doing drugs. AIDS wasn't a part of my life."

In time, he stopped kidding myself and got diagnosed. Everything seemed to fall apart. Okay. I'm positive now. Fuck the career, he thought. A computer hacker, Teddy could have earned big bucks, but it was never his nature "to think of pension plans." Convinced death was imminent, he gave up.

Sitting in the hospital bed, a white rat for AIDS research, Teddy's natural character had returned. "I will not be on that quilt," he said, referring to the AIDS quilt made up of thousands of panels, each representing a death from AIDS. "I will not be a panel on that quilt."

He thought his attitude arrogant but logical. "There are just too many drugs out there. There will be a cure out there soon. I do feel sorry for the early people. There was just nothing they could do. I'm lucky I guess."

Lunch trays were brought in at noon. Teddy traded Harold a tuna sandwich for a ham. Two years ago to the week, Teddy had been diagnosed. He want to Ward 86 in the old brick building. A week later he was started on one of the General's drug trials. It gave him a shooting pain but he got over it. "You know pain. The day after it's over, it's like it never happened." So he went on another drug protocol: Both drugs were, as he put it, "a bust." Yet that did not lessen his desire to go on Q, his third drug trial.

"You may as well deal with this disease aggressively," he explained. "It's not the thrill of my life, but it's better than sitting back."

Teddy would probably have quit partying anyway. "At around twenty-five your priorities are supposed to start changing. . . . AIDS was just another reason." Recently Teddy had started feeling grown-up. "I'm finally an adult. I'm acting like all the other adults," he said, with a childlike grin.

"Hi. I've had all my Compound Q. I'm not comatose and I'm fine." Harold was calling his boyfriend with the news. "I'm in here for twenty-four hours. In case something happens. They can watch.

"I have a cute roommate. You'd definitely recognize him. He's from the circuit."

Then Harold and Teddy talked about Muscle Systems and how dedicated they had to be to keep up the regime. Sometimes, they said, they overdo it. "A lot of gay men are very physicalistic," Teddy said. He didn't want to get to the point where he'd only go out with men whose muscles are of a certain size.

Many of the clubs of the gay heyday had closed (Trocadero was still open), but the gyms lived on. Harold and Teddy still met nice men. Harold would only go out with other HIV-positive men, and there were plenty of those to go around. Teddy played a little looser. "If someone is positive, what are you supposed to do" Harold asked. "Fold up your sex life?"

"I almost feel sorry for gay men who are negative," said the effervescent Teddy. His thinking may be delusional, but it suited him. "I was so relieved when I found out I was positive," he declared. "The stress was gone."

That night, the blondes visited. Teddy's boyfriend got into bed with him. When a nurse walked in she found Teddy on top. "You're not supposed to be doing that in here," she said. Teddy and the blonde retired to the lounge. There, Teddy lay on his friend's chest. Another nice nurse advised: "I know you're happy, but you have to be a little more discreet."

That night Harold felt fine. Teddy got a case of the Q flu. He had the chills and felt very tired. Heartburn bothered him. He asked for another blanket and blamed the heartburn on hospital food.

The Bad Dream

The well-groomed, lanky black woman with a cut, broken nose approached the nursing station of the emergency room. Turning to medical student Melissa Bartick and the house staff, she politely inquired if she might use the phone. It was 4 A.M.

"Mama," she said on making the call, "we got in a big fight. I pushed him. He punched me in the nose, so I took out the butcher knife and I stabbed him in the chest a couple of times and then I stabbed him in the stomach."

Melissa and the others couldn't help but hear.

"I told him 'You wimp! You pussy!' And I kicked him and said 'You're bleeding on my floor. Get up. I'm going to the hospital.'"

"Yeah, Mom. It was bad."

The conversation ended. The woman smiled in a most civil way, apologizing for tying up the phone. "But you know how it is when you're talking to your mother."

For a middle-class medical student, the culture of violence was at the same time appalling and fascinating. Many of Melissa's patients lived lives at risk. At times, she, too, was taking risks. But part of the job, as Melissa saw it, was helping "the underserved." Not even a knife-wielding woman with a wimp for a boyfriend could deter Melissa. Besides, she had a duty to see all patients.

In the treatment room, Melissa inquired about the stabbing. Although she seemed to be a "nice" person, the woman appeared unconcerned about her victim.

Melissa wouldn't give up.

"What kind of knife did you use?

"A butcher knife."

"How big was it?"

"Oh, I got one just like it in my purse," the woman said with equanimity, pulling out a butcher knife as if it were a snapshot of the kids.

"Don't get that thing near me," Melissa warned.

"Oh, I don't stab women," the patient reassured. "I just beat them up."

While Melissa cleaned her patient's nose, the woman chatted affably about the man she'd stabbed.

Only the other week some woman came knocking on her door saying, "What are you doing with my husband?"

"What? Rodney's married?" the patient had said.

"I'm Rodney's wife."

The patient had beat up the wife.

"Did you see her?" she asked Melissa. "Veronica. It would have been Wednesday night she came in here."

Melissa asked how far the knife plunged into her boyfriend's chest and stomach. The woman stretched her hands apart about four inches.

"You know you could have killed him," Melissa said.

"Yeah," the patient replied. "You're trying to make me feel guilty."

"Did you want to kill him?"

"I didn't care. I just wanted to hurt him."

"You know you could be charged with murder and get life in prison," Melissa advised.

"I didn't think about that."

Afraid of needles, the woman refused to have her nose stitched. Melissa taped it instead. Despite the violence, the bloody nose and the long knife in the patient's purse, Melissa couldn't help but enjoy the woman.

Although she's liberal, Melissa did not think that all poor people are good people who haven't had a chance. At the General, she'd seen plenty of "jerks." Some resented her white coat, her mantle of authority. Others ordered her around, yelled and brought her to tears. Still, she tried to teach them about living healthy lives.

A Caucasian patient with a likable personality and a life destroyed had come to the hospital complaining of abdominal pain from PID: pelvic inflammatory disease. An IV drug user, crack addict and sexual partner to numerous men, her children had been taken from her. Recently, she'd given birth to another and because of her addiction, that baby, too, had been taken away.

As Melissa took the woman's blood, she asked about a scar on her arm.

"I give plasma," the woman said.

"You give plasma?" Melissa said incredulously. Given the woman's history, Melissa knew there was a good chance she was HIV positive. She was just the kind of high-risk person the plasma and blood banks were trying to screen out to keep the blood supply safe. (Sometime after this incident, Melissa learned that paid plasma is used for research.)

"What do you do when they ask you if you shoot drugs?"

"I just lie and tell them I don't."

"You could kill somebody," Melissa said in her quiet manner. "If I were you, I would find another way to make money."

The patient was outraged. "I didn't come here for you to tell me how to live my life!" she screamed. "I came here for treatment! I didn't come here to listen to this shit!"

She threatened to put on her clothes and stomp out.

Dressed and pacing the corridors, she shouted, "I hope the bitch loses her job!"

The woman continued to shout her complaints and, in the process, forgot her pain.

"You're only mad because you know it's true," Melissa said.

The woman stayed for treatment.

No matter how harshly the few truly difficult patients behaved toward Melissa, she continued to try to educate them about AIDS.

Scary moments occurred when Melissa was rotating through the emergency room. One night, a suicidal woman was brought in an ambulance after ingesting a large amount of heroin and alcohol. She didn't want to be at the hospital and she didn't want to cooperate. She said she was HIV positive. She lay on a gurney with an IV in her arm.

Savvy about hospital policy, she asked to use the phone by the nursing station. Rising from the gurney, she trailed the IV bag with her. As she was talking on the phone, she pulled out her IV. Blood splattered everywhere—onto sweaters, jackets, chairs and the floor. The patient didn't care. She had greater concerns: her boyfriend had been fooling around with her sister.

Put back on the gurney, she was placed in four-point restraints. The confinement angered her.

"You could have killed somebody," said Melissa, who wasn't really angry. She just thought being direct and confrontational would be more effective.

"Well," the patient replied, "everyone's going to die of AIDS anyway."

The woman had only learned recently that she was HIV positive. She hadn't yet told her boyfriend. "I still can't believe it myself," she said. Another sister (not the one who had stolen the boyfriend) and a brother-in-law were also HIV positive. In the patient's world, Melissa figured, she might be right that everyone would die of AIDS.

Melissa counseled, "No matter what your boyfriend did, you have to tell him soon."

"I'll work on it," the woman said.

While the woman was in restraints, Melissa had to get an arterial blood gas test. A heavy smoker and asthmatic, the woman's oxygen saturation was low. Melissa had to find out why. Because the patient was HIV positive, the procedure could be dangerous. Melissa wasn't really thinking about the risk, she was just thinking that the woman needed the test. Melissa reached for the patient's wrist, the standard place to draw the sample. Covered with a lambswool restraint, there remained little space for the medical student to place her fingers. Melissa could have gone to the groin. She could have called a nurse to help. She didn't think about it. A vein is visible. An artery is harder to locate. The walls of the artery are thicker so the blood can't be seen at the surface. Melissa felt for a pulse in each finger. She imagined the location of the artery between the two fingers. If she hit a vein, the blood would ooze; hit an artery and the blood would shoot up. Melissa warned the patient the procedure would hurt. She plunged the needle in. Despite the restraints, the woman jumped. The needle popped out, nearly hitting Melissa's finger.

Melissa immediately called for a nurse. The nurse told her she should get the blood gas by the brachial artery, along the inside of the arm, near the woman's elbow, which can cause more complications for the patient but in this case, was safer for the medical staff.

This was not the first time that Melissa's inexperience put her at risk. Maybe, she thought, I'm one of those people who's just denying the danger. She knew people who'd been stuck with needles full of HIV-positive blood. "One of these days. I might. I know that. I kind of have this attitude that you can't let fears run your life. . . . If I get stuck, if I change and become positive, I guess that's just what will happen. That's just what will happen with my life, how my life will end."

When Melissa had applied to medical school in 1984, AIDS was an isolated disease. She knew that Haitians got it, and she didn't know any Haitians. Her fear there may have been an oversupply of doctors and her fear of not being able to find a job were at least as prominent as her concern about AIDS.

"I never thought of it as directly threatening me. Yeah, I'd heard of it. [But] I didn't know it was going to be an epidemic. I didn't know it was going to be in San Francisco. I think even if I'd known, it wouldn't have stopped me.

"I suppose if I'd come from Vermont this would be scary for me here. But it's not how my life worked out. That's okay."

While working on the east side of the emergency room—for patients who'd been stabbed or cut, had broken bones or had been in accidents, Melissa was amazed by their gory injuries and stories of unprovoked violence.

A gay man from her Castro district neighborhood was brought in after being beaten with a lead pipe and sticks by a gang of Spanish-speaking kids. Due to the language barrier, the gay patient never knew for certain why he had been a target, but since he hadn't been robbed, he assumed it was an act of gay bashing. His head bled profusely from the pummeling he received.

A few hours later, another victim of another beating arrived in the ER. He and a friend had been driving through a public housing project.

While halted at a stop sign, they had been pulled out of their car by what he believed to be a gang of Samoans. He also suffered scalp lacerations.

Melissa saw a lot of drunken patients injured in fights over women. Sometimes she cared for patients under police guards. One with whom she developed a rapport was under arrest for murder. Drunk but laughing, the patient joked with Melissa while she stitched up his arm. "I don't pass judgment on what they allegedly did," Melissa explained. "I wasn't there. I don't know the circumstances. Besides, that's not my place to pass judgment in any case."

Each time, before sewing up a patient's wound, Melissa had to irrigate the area to clean it out. The procedure involved hanging a bag of saline solution and, with the help of gravity, squirting the liquid into the wound.

When Melissa irrigated the bloody wounds in the ER, the solution and blood splashed on her. The first few times she forgot to wear goggles, standard equipment in the era of AIDS. The patient's blood easily could have splattered into her eyes. AIDS can be transmitted when HIV-positive blood comes in contact with the mucous membrane of the eye, nose or mouth. Even when Melissa remembered to put on goggles she was at risk. Her head was so small that she needed child-size goggles. Those provided by the hospital slid off. Eventually, Melissa got in the habit of taping the goggles to fit.

She knew she had to be conscientious. Practicing medicine, she felt, "was like playing music." Melissa played the violin. "You have to attend to every note. You can't even for a minute let your mind lapse."

The close calls, exposure to violence and the presence of the AIDS virus were playing on her psyche. Melissa had a dream in which she was HIV positive. Her whole life changed. "I found out I was positive and I was regretting the very day I found out. It wasn't the typical thing where you say: 'My days are numbered. I should go and have fun.'" Because consciously, she knew that if she faced a life sentence, she "sure wouldn't spend it in medical school."

In the dream she tried to "forget about the day I learned I was positive. . . . I tried for a time to give myself relief of not knowing and [the chance] to live freely as I had before. And I couldn't wipe it from the back of my mind. Always lingering there was that I was positive. Those were like days of freedom and this was almost like slavery. This knowledge.

"I kept telling myself, 'This is just your fate. This is how your life is going to go. Some people live to be old but you won't. This is what God wants.' But I couldn't believe it. I would tell myself that but it only brought superficial comfort."

The effects of the dream were long lasting. Her innocence and sense of invulnerability were shot. "In my dream, I had to live through years of doom before I even would have years of being sick, having dementia and wasting away.

"I used to feel that AIDS patients should be treated like any other patients," Melissa said. "Now I don't think so." She didn't believe that doctors should pick and choose procedures at will but she thought that they should include a patient's HIV status when weighing cases where the procedure is not 100 percent necessary for the patient's health.

She used to feel that the statistics on needle-stick seroconversion were "very low." Not anymore. "If you're the one [who acquires HIV on the job], your risk of dying is 100 percent."

Still HIV Positive

I'm still HIV positive."

The first two years after the accident had been "the golden days." Back then, thoughts of the virus were episodic. Now, they were nearly constant.

Jane Doe found it easier to deal with bedridden AIDS patients at the hospital than to care for those barely ambulatory, like the emaciated men still in street clothes, trying to live their lives outside the hospital. To look at them was to see the progression of the disease, the slow ebbing of energy, the loss of appetite, the body drained. She couldn't help but wonder, Is this what I'm in for? Only she didn't say it. In soft, caring tones, she'd console the patients. She couldn't express the subtext. Because what she really wanted to do was jump on the furniture and yell. She wanted to pick up a bottle and throw it against the wall.

At twenty-seven, Jane Doe wasn't like the legions of gay men in San Francisco who went to more funerals than their grandparents did. Nothing had prepared her for this.

For the most part, Jane Doe was optimistic. She believed she could beat AIDS. Her timing was good. She believed she'd live long enough for there to be a cure and if not a cure, a drug that made AIDS a chronic disease like diabetes.

Sometimes Jane Doe wanted to rush up to Dr. McGrath, the discoverer of Q, and thank him. Other times she felt the pace of research excruciatingly slow. Slow for her. Slow for a friend starting to show symptoms of AIDS. Jane Doe wondered if, when her friend became deathly sick, she might be prompted to knock down doors and yell, "Give me that Compound Q this minute!" McGrath and Dr. Volberding were married men. They had no risk, no clock, no major threat that they knew about. The fact was that all during the epidemic, a whole lot of HIV-negative people had been making decisions for HIV-positive people. That's what happened when Jane Doe asked the city to preserve her privacy. And that, she felt, was what was happening in medicine, too.

Jane Doe sounded like an activist with Project Inform or ACT UP, groups she respected. But she felt too weary to become involved. Stress wasn't good for someone with the virus. And sometimes she just needed to focus on having a regular life. She needed to go out to dinner, read a book, laugh or sit in the tub. She needed, she said, to take care of her immune system.

Medical advice, she left to her doctors. Anxious to know if she should take AZT, she sought out the expert, Volberding.

Struck by his warmth and empathetic eyes, she sensed an immediate rapport. Dispensing with AIDS 101, he treated her like a professional. He'd asked her to bring her numbers. In preparation, she'd drawn a graph. He drew the slope. When a person's T4 cell count dropped to 500 it was recommended he be put on AZT. When it dropped to 200, doctors often put a patient on aerosol pentamidine to stave off AIDS pneumonia. Jane Doe felt her numbers were good. Volberding was interested in the slope. For the first time, Jane Doe realized that her immune cells were dropping. At 800, her T4 cell count was still high. But the slope showed she'd lost a quarter of the critical cells.

Volberding and the nurse talked rationally about her numbers and available medicines. They discussed AZT. Jane Doe felt that what they were really talking about was whether she would live to be thirty-two or thirty-five. The rational part of her felt grounded, present, engaged. The emotional part wanted to leap onto his desk and scream, "Isn't this outrageous? Isn't this totally outrageous that anybody should have to go through this? Isn't this horrible? Can you imagine having fifty years cut off your life?" She didn't and he didn't. In his calm demeanor, Jane Doe understood that Volberding's life was safer, which was how hers used to be, too. Most doctors and nurses, like most of the rest of the population, felt immune. That was the only way they could look at and care for patients suffering from such an atrocity. In the midst of that security, Jane Doe felt quite alone, even among friends.

She found it much easier to date medical people, but she couldn't always limit herself. Nonmedical people were so scared. "People are out there fucking their brains out," she said, "using safe sex and believing in safe sex, believing in the scientific basis of safe sex. Then they come up against an HIV-positive person and suddenly, safe sex is no longer scientific."

Too often, Jane Doe felt herself pulled into the role of girlfriend and educator. "I've had to tell my lovers, You need to educate yourself. I can't feel like I'm the one trying to persuade you to take a risk with me. I can't."

One boyfriend had reservations about dating her because she probably would never have children. "People fall in love with people who can't have children," Jane Doe told him. In anger, she asked, "Have you had a sperm count? Are you going to have your beloved checked for fertility before you marry her? How do you know you're not going to end up in the exact situation you're trying so hard to avoid? This is life," she said, echoing her mother's words. "This is what happens."

She was angry, not just at the boyfriend, not just at the situation, but at her loss. "It isn't just about children or dating," she said. "It's about feeling so incredibly different, feeling so stripped of so many of the illusions that are luxuries for other people." They assumed they would marry, have kids and life would end happily ever after. Jane Doe no longer shared in those assumptions.

With her warmth, smarts and good looks, men were attracted to her. One night, when she was locked out of her apartment, she decided to go to the hospital to sleep. She called a cab to take her to Potrero Hill, the neighborhood that houses the General. A friendly, nice driver, the cabbie said he'd been reading about the nurse who stuck herself and seroconverted. He asked, "Do you know whatever happened to that person?"

There was a long pause. Jane Doe had a good gut feeling about him, so she did something that was totally out of character. His head turned toward the backseat. With a smile and a twinkle, Jane Doe said, "Hello." The cabbie was in shock. They pulled into the emergency-room parking lot. He said she'd had a rough night. He suggested she pay only half fare. She insisted on paying full. He wanted to buy her coffee sometime. She said fine. For five weeks, they followed the modern American dating ritual, each one talking to the other's answering machine. Eventually they went to the beach on a date. They walked along. They kissed. And he said, "You never know what's going to go on in your life. You read about a person in the paper and then you're kissing her on the beach."

The two became involved. From the cabbie and from other friends, Jane Doe sought support, believing she could survive AIDS. Sometimes friends slipped up. To one friend, Jane Doe had described her visits East, to see her parents. "They treat me like gold," she'd marveled. Jane Doe didn't bother adding that they treat her brother that way, too, because, she explained later, both live three thousand miles away from home. Without realizing how hopeless it sounded, the friend said, "Well, they're aware of time."

Jane Doe was trying to be good to herself. She often felt fury at no one in particular. If only she could buy cheap cases of Woolworth's glassware and live in a two-bedroom apartment—one for sleeping, the other for throwing glass—then she thought she'd feel better.

Trying to avoid obsessive thoughts of AIDS, attempting to bypass her rational mind, she was dipping into massage and dance and a small amount of spirituality, all of which was a little hard. Sometimes she needed to remind her instructors that she was from the East Coast. Regularly she put on her Walkman and rode the bus downtown to the Y to attend aerobics classes. And she watched what she ate, most of the time.

Occasionally, she'd stop by a fast-food store. "Oh, my God," she marveled at a sausage-egg-and-cheese sandwich, "this garbage is so good!" A lot of HIV-positive people diligently care for themselves, observing stringent diets and building up their bodies. One of Jane Doe's close friends had a different attitude. He'd seen more guys come into the General in beautiful shape on special diets, drinking only bottled water. And he saw them die. As far as he was concerned, he told Jane Doe, "I'm eating Cheese Doodles the rest of my life."

Jane Doe wanted to exercise, eat right and meditate. And she wanted to believe that that would guarantee her survival. "I know it can't. I like quick answers. And I like guarantees. If I do this . . . I want it signed, sealed and delivered." That told Jane Doe something: "That I still carry around this basic denial."

Jane Doe continued to work at the General. Nurses and doctors there were a lot more careful about needles and blood splashes than they'd been before she stuck herself. But little else seemed to change. Hospital administrators had promised to put red Sharps boxes, used to dispose of dirty needles, closer to patients' bedsides. Nearly three years later, the hospital was preparing to install new Sharps boxes on the wall above patients' beds.

It tore at Jane Doe to know that a safer needle had been available at the time of her accident but that the General and other hospitals had found it too costly. Administrators worried that to buy safe needles the hospital budget for such items might go from seven hundred thousand dollars annually to seven million. "We're looking for the maximum amount of safety within our budgetary constraints," said Phillip Sowa, then executive director at the General.

Jane Doe despised Dr. Day's attitude toward AIDS patients. She once heard Day on the radio, warning people against protected sex with HIV-positive partners. Hadn't Day already caused enough problems, Jane Doe thought. Bringing attention to safety issues was important, Jane Doe agreed, but she felt Day "was generating paranoia and that her arguments were not without homophobia."

Three years after Jane Doe stuck herself, the General, which is more progressive than most hospitals, was still using the brand of needle that Jane Doe had used. It had begun to evaluate safer needles.

Four Out of Seven Beds

The ambulance doors swung open. "Hang loose, man. We're here to help you out and see the doctors." The paramedic leaned over the gurney. "Hang in there." They flipped down the metal legs of the gurney as they lowered it to street level.

Blood covered most of the man's head and face. He wore an oxygen mask. A gauze beret the paramedics had made for him was soaked a dark red. Blood poured down the man's chest. "*Open your eyes, man! Stay with it!*" the paramedic yelled as they wheeled him into the hospital and down the corridor.

"Two stab wounds left lower thorax, multiple stab wounds to the head," called a paramedic as they entered the trauma room.

While riding the bus shortly after 2 A.M., three men had attacked him with knives. "Assailants unknown," the paramedic called, using starched police lingo. By the time the ambulance had arrived, the bus was awash in blood.

Ten doctors and nurses, some with goggles, all with gloves, stood over the silent patient. Simultaneously they checked the ABC's of the emergency room: airways, breathing and circulation. Through observation, they could see his chest rise and fall. With two fingers to the carotid artery at his neck, a nurse checked his pulse. Another nurse shoved an IV into his arm. Before hooking him up to a solution, she drew blood and sent it to the lab to check his blood chemistry, electrolytes, kidney and liver functions. The lab would determine his blood type so that units of blood could be reserved in case he required surgery. A mask was clamped over his mouth and nose to give him oxygen.

When someone pushed a catheter up the patient's penis, he came to: "*What are you doing?*" he screamed. "*Stop it!*"

"We need to do it to see if you're bleeding down there," someone said.

"Stop doing it down there! Please!" he begged.

"It's done. Just relax."

Nurses, wiping blood off his back, looked for more stab wounds. Puddles of blood sat on the brown stretcher.

Everyone in the trauma room but the patient ran into the hallway as a chest X ray hurriedly was taken. Doctors needed to scan his lungs for puncture wounds. When they ran back, Tom, the primary nurse, inquired, "What bus line was that? Remind me to stay off that." Throughout the evening, the nurse with the puckish humor tried to inject levity into somber settings.

"Let me call your mom or your dad," he said to the patient.

Through the oxygen mask came a muffled no.

"Let me call someone else."

"No."

On one gurney or another rested all the problems of urban America: violence, AIDS, homelessness, alcoholism, drugs, and nearly every disease medical students have read about. Attending physician Dr. Gerald Hill had come to expect the emergency room drama. Late one Saturday night, four out of the seven ER beds were filled with AIDS patients or those suspected of having HIV-related problems. About half the AIDS patients admitted to the hospital come to the side entrance on the first floor of the gray main building, or what Hill endearingly called "this wacko, crazy environment."

At this the port of entry, many men barely out of their teens learned that they had the AIDS virus. Many arrived with hacking coughs. The first thing Hill considered was PCP, the pneumonia associated with

AIDS. At most hospitals around the country, Hill wouldn't dare ask someone if he was gay or straight, but at the General, he had to.

Here in the ER, nurses had no time for hand holding, back rubbing or empathetic conversations that characterize the AIDS care in Ward 86 (the outpatient unit down the block) and 5A (the inpatient unit five floors up). Everything in the emergency room was threateningly fast. There were almost always too many patients and not enough staff or space. Sometimes patients, of unknown HIV status, would kick, bite and splatter their blood. The ER was a high-risk environment for health-care workers where the only certainty was the chaos.

"Where do you live?" resident Michon Morita asked a sickly looking woman in pink kerchief whose head barely poked out above the thermal blanket.

"Nowhere," she said. A brown paper bag full of her possessions and a pair of sneakers were parked on the lower shelf of her gurney.

"Have you used IV drugs at all?" he asked.

"I used to."

Nearly every time he drew blood, Morita considered the risks. Even when he took all the precautions, he figured, "It's still dangerous."

"It's like the substance that is common to all of us," said one hospital nurse, "is now deadly." She was talking about blood.

Morita drew the patient's blood to check for bacterial pneumonia, although he thought it more likely that she had Pneumocystis carinii pneumonia.

"She's probably been exposed to the AIDS virus," he said, placing the needle in the red Sharps box on the wall.

Because she was homeless, she would be admitted. Alone, she might not take her medication or show up for her checkup. "We'll keep her from dying out in the streets," he said.

When Morita brought the woman's X rays to the radiologist who could determine what kind of pneumonia she had, the younger doctor told the radiologist, "She's had a fever, cough, pretty normal lung exam. And, oh yeah, she might be HIV positive."

"Around here," said the radiologist, "that comes first. Either that or we just assume it."

Morita had gone to medical school in St. Louis, where AIDS was only one of many diseases. Here at the General it was never far from his mind. "A lot of the public is down on the medical community for being so concerned with their health," he said. "But think about it, someone my age who doesn't drink, doesn't smoke and doesn't belong to a gang. There aren't many reasons for me to die in my twenties."

Ward 86 and the inpatient AIDS ward were both controlled environments. Nothing, it seemed, was ever under control in the ER.

Along with the mix of HIV-positive patients and the man stabbed on the bus was an inmate from the county jail. His head was collapsed on a table, his legs in metal restraints hooked to his chair. He wore peach-colored wool socks and, on his face, a grimace. Periodically he moaned, complaining of abdominal pain. When dinner arrived, he chowed down the lasagna, the roll and everything else. An "impressive appetite," Hill remarked, and it made him wonder about the veracity of the patient's complaints. "It's either San Francisco General or the jail."

A savvy physician, Hill was wearing tennis shoes, jeans, shirt, tie and white jacket. Only when he turned away did the complexity of the man become obvious.; A long ponytail trailed down half his back. He's a Klamath Indian from Klamath Falls, Oregon, who's sculpted a place for himself at the hospital. His work is devoted to indigent care. In his free time he works on Indian health care. When he began medical school in 1976 there were only forty-five American Indian doctors in the United States. Today, Hill is president of the Association of American Indian Physicians, which has two hundred members. According to the United States 1990 census, there are now twice that number practicing. Hill attributes the increase to Indian activism of the '60s and '70s.

"Please telephone my lover, Joseph," said a young man with dyed yellow hair that stood straight up like that of a surprised comic-book character. "I just love him," he giggled. A nurse named Ann rolled her eyes and obliged. She had the tolerance of a harried waitress at a busy New York deli. He'd come in with a seizure, the result of not taking his Dilantin, the drug which controlled the seizures caused by his HIV-crippled nervous system.

Even after learning that Joseph was at home, the patient shouted to the table of doctors nearby, "I'm better off not being released." He wanted to be admitted but he wasn't even close.

For twenty minutes, Morita stayed with the patient, giving him his Dilantin and checking his blood pressure. For twenty minutes he listened to the patient's ramblings about his present lover and his past ones. The patient loudly confided to the resident, "I have ARC. I always use safe sex because I'm afraid I might get AIDS." Morita didn't know quite what to say. The patient already had the AIDS virus.

While the night was still slow, Hill and the residents and interns huddled around a small table telling medical war stories. They spoke fondly of James, a homeless alcoholic with a kindly disposition, frequently picked up "frozen solid, cold and drunk," carted to the General, patched up and released. A lot of drunks are cantakerous; not James. He wouldn't even urinate in front of a woman doctor. "He's very humble, very polite and just a total loss to humanity," said Leda Felicio, a first-year medical resident. The previous week, James had come through the emergency room three times with what the medical staff said was the body temperature the level of antifreeze. He had been found in front of a Burger King with a Whopper in his hand and maggots on his body.

"He's an American Indian from Minnesota," Hill told them. Several times, Hill had sent James to an alcoholism program specifically designed for Indians. Always, James returned to the General.

Throughout the hospital, but especially in the ER, patients of all ethnicities come. So it's ironic that an oil painting, hung upstairs near the hospital cafeteria, depicted doctors, nurses and orderlies of all races crowded around an idealized bedridden blond, blue-eyed woman. Hill had always disliked the picture. To him, it implied that the typical General patient, who most certainly was not shown in the painting, wasn't worth it. And he thought that if the hospital artwork were accurate, the patient would be a minority-group member with AIDS.

Hill wished there were more minority nurses and doctors in ER. Patients were more willing to open up to those with whom they shared a culture. And he believed that history was 90 percent of medicine.

A fifty-year-old American Indian woman was brought into ER one night drunk. She fell off her gurney and the nurse put her back on. She fell off a second time. The nurse put her back on again and yelled that if she fell off again, the patient would be thrown out of the emergency room. The nurse was shocked when Hill told him the patient was his cousin.

Born on a reservation, Hill had left after his parents' divorce—the result of alcohol and family violence. Not until he met an Indian medical student did he consider becoming a physician. After medical school at the University of Washington in Seattle and residency at UCSF, he participated in the prestigious Robert Wood Johnson Clinical

Scholars Program. But when he applied for a position at Stanford University Medical School, he felt he was discriminated against. Someone less qualified than he got the job. An official at Stanford, whose mascot had been the Stanford Indian, told him that he didn't get the job because they were concerned that he "wouldn't be happy there."

"I'm calling Joseph," Ann said to the yellow-haired patient.

"I just love him," the patient shouted back.

"Joseph. Did I wake you up? This is Ann again at General. We're going to be releasing him in about ten or fifteen minutes or so."

When she returned to the patient, he kiddingly requested "mountain spring water." If that wasn't available, he'd settle for just plain water. His IV removed, the patient wouldn't budge. Sitting upright in his bed, wearing his blue-and-white hospital gown, he said, "Can I have some clothes to wear home?" He'd soiled the clothes he came in. In anticipation of such situations, the hospital maintains a supply of secondhand clothes.

"I can't find my shoes," he said, stalling for time. Someone had brought him a soccer T-shirt and pants but no shoes. "I wear size thirteen," he declared.

A nurse trotted off to find size thirteen.

"These shoes are too small," he complained.

She went back to find another pair. The second pair, he contended, slipped off.

"This isn't Thom McAn," said the exasperated nurse.

In another bed lay a rickety thin woman. She said she was an alcoholic and claimed no longer to use heroin. She'd come in with abcesses. When she tottered to the bathroom, she lugged her purse along. "She probably just shot up," a doctor said. "We gave her Valium for her alcohol withdrawal, and she probably took care of the other."

In another bed a polite old Asian woman complained to Morita that her stomach hurt and she had chest pains. She seemed out of place. With all the cases of drug addicts and AIDS patients the old woman received little attention.

Someone spilled the metal wastebasket in the room. Used white gloves, sleeves from syringes and papers spilled onto the floor. Nobody knelt down to clean it up. By mistake, someone might have dumped a used needle into the garbage. Housekeeping was called.

A homeless woman having seizures, a male alcoholic and a patient who had tried to kill himself with barbiturates were brought in.

What had begun as a slow Saturday night was speeding up and spinning out of control. The table where the doctors and nurses had huddled was now empty.

In the trauma part of the emergency room was a man who had been shot in the eye with a pellet gun. Another had been in an auto accident. Someone had fallen off his motorbike and another man had been assaulted with a baseball bat. Another had been stabbed in the back three times. A sailor had fallen or jumped four stories. A pool player had been stabbed by a pool cue.

The stabbing victim had his oxygen mask removed so he could throw up. Hill and others wore blue plastic aprons. The patient's oxygen mask was replaced. Blood coated his torso.

"Who would you like me to call?" Nurse Tom asked.

"Nobody."

"You don't have anybody? Maybe you'll meet a nice nurse upstairs."

A white sheet covering the mat above the gurney was soaked in blood.

The stabbing victim's lung had collapsed. Doctors made an incision between his ribs and inserted a chest tube into his pleural space to pull air out, equalizing the pressure so that his lung could expand.

"Just squeeze my hand," a woman doctor told the patient. Instantly he complied. Squeezing diverted attention from the pain. When the doctor went on to other chores, the patient's left arm kept reaching out to the air, his fingers flopping up and down in search of a hand no longer there.

Elsewhere in the ER the sickest AIDS patient of the night could barely move. Like many, he'd tried to manage on his own for as long as he could. Four months before, he'd been in the emergency room with PCP. That was when he learned he was HIV positive. He was beginning to waste away. Once again, he had trouble breathing, fever and chills. Lisa Adams, a fourth-year Dartmouth medical student visiting San Francisco General's ER for a month, examined him. She'd spent ten months in medicine in Hanover, New Hampshire, and seen only one AIDS patient. When she drew this man's blood she couldn't help but think it was deadly. The thought overwhelmed her.

In the rush of the moment, the very sick AIDS patient was just one of a half dozen patients needing immediate attention.

Nurse Tom passed another nurse: "When you get to the door lock it, for Christ's sake," he said.

In the hallway, the man beaten with a baseball bat waited for attention. He complained of chest pains and left-flank pain and he competitively claimed he had the worst injury of the night.

The pool-cue victim requested a mirror to study his blemished face and head.

Two police officers interviewed the pool-cue patient in the hallway.

"Do you know who won the game?" the pool-playing patient inquired.

"What game?"

"The pool game," he replied.

The man with the drug overdose had been given charcoal to absorb the drug and medication to induce vomiting. A worried medical student in a blue apron moved the patient's body to redirect the projectile vomiting away from other people. Already bloodied on his face and hands, the charcoal that came up spilled black fluid all over the patient. In wonderment, he inspected his left hand, compared it to that of the black patient in the bed next to him and laughed: "I'm black like you!" The black patient was in too much pain to hear.

A janitor came through with a broom, sweeping the mess on the floor out of the room. In amongst the used white gloves and papers a dime glimmered. No one picked it up.

No Right Answers

On this cold January day, four patients in the respiratory intensive care unit had Pneumocystis carinii pneumonia (PCP), the most common of AIDS opportunistic infections. All of them were on mechanized ventilators. A fifth patient, a resident of Civic Center plaza, came in badly beaten. With swollen lymph nodes and a history of drug use, it was assumed he was HIV positive. The sixth patient, an eighty-five-year-old Filipino, had viral pneumonia.

The comatose Mr. Davis, one of the PCP patients, lay tethered to life. A pink bag of sugar water was infused into a feeding tube that tunneled through his nostril to his stomach; an IV fed him antibiotics. Another tube passed through his windpipe, allowing him to breathe on a mechanical ventilator. A yellowish arterial catheter inserted into an artery in his wrist measured his blood pressure and allowed physicians to draw blood gases painlessly to measure the oxygen in his blood. Two tubes went into his chest, one of which reached the lining of his lung to prevent the lung from collapsing. Leads were pasted onto his chest to permit electrocardiographic monitoring. A Foley catheter snaked through his penis to his bladder. His feet were in splints, forced into a neutral position so they couldn't contract from disuse. With a loud, swishing sound, the ventilator pumped air into his lungs.

Mr. Davis represented the new breed. An IV drug user, he'd come to the emergency room complaining of a fever, not knowing he had AIDS. Like an insecure teenager, he attached himself to resident Mark Tonelli, who found the patient genuinely likable. When Mr. Davis learned he had AIDS, he grew terrified and failed to appear for an appointment at the General. Because he'd given his name as Mr. Poirot (he was said to be hiding from drug dealers) and a wrong address, he could not be reached.

The next time Tonelli saw the patient he'd been dumped off at the emergency room by "a friend." Mr. Davis was having trouble breathing. When resident Tonelli reached the ER, Mr. Davis was already on a ventilator.

He was the first patient the residents and intensive-care doctor John Luce examined on their morning rounds. From the beginning of the epidemic, former chief of staff Luce had been involved. Now he was facing complex ethical issues about life and how long a physician should insist it be continued.

"We ended up deciding he was a twenty-seven-year-old with AIDS," Tonelli said, running down his case to the medical team. By then, Mr. Davis had been hooked up to a ventilator for thirty-one days, a length of time that aroused concern.

Twice, Tonelli had lowered Mr. Davis's sedatives and morphine to ask him if he wanted to continue on the ventilator. The physician warned his patient his lungs weren't going to get any better and it wasn't likely he'd ever get off the tube. Tonelli asked the patient if he wanted to continue. Both times, Mr. Davis thrashed about, his eyes bulged, and he said yes. The doctor could tell that "as miserable as it was to live on the ventilator, he still didn't want to die."

Tonelli and the other residents recognized the right of a patient to determine his own medical care. They also understood the most basic principle in medical ethics: beneficence—benefiting the patient by relieving pain, treating illness and sustaining life.

Including hospital expenses, equipment and nursing, it cost at least twenty-eight hundred dollars per day to keep Mr. Davis in the intensive care unit, not counting doctor fees. There are always more seriously ill patients than there are beds or ventilators available.

It had been clear to resident Juliana Matthews from the first day she'd seen the patient that he wasn't going to survive. It was probably clear to everyone involved in his case—everyone but Mr. Davis and Mr. Davis's God-fearing mother.

"So he's basically stuck in this position?" a female resident inquired.

"You're stuck in this position because no one has ever forced the issue in a public way. So there's no law," said Luce, associate director of the medical-surgical intensive care unit and associate professor in medicine and anesthesia at UC Med Center.

Luce told the assembled doctors that if the therapy was futile they could stop it. But, he warned, the family could take them to court.

The house staff moved from room to room, studying the young men kept alive by machinery. When Luce had been in training, such issues were never discussed. Medical care was considered a right. These new doctors, living in an era of tighter money and greater technology, longed for some social policy to help direct them.

"Do you have any experience if they turn around, like, what day it might be?" a resident asked.

Luce couldn't predict. There was nothing identifiable in the patients that indicated who was going to get better and who wasn't.

"Some people get better after fourteen days, after twenty-one days of therapy, so you couldn't just allow a week as a clinical trial. . . . If you're serious about it, you have to give it more time. What the upper limits are is unclear."

Troubled by the issue, Luce earlier had asked for advice from his weekly meeting with other chest doctors from various San Francisco hospitals. He sought "some kind of group thought as to what an adequate trial on a mechanical ventilator" might be for AIDS patients. He knew everyone would equivocate, and everyone did. He pushed some more: "It would be nice if we had some kind of internal consistency so we can tell the house staff." It depended on the patient, they said. A physician cited the case of a deathly ill PCP patient who remained on the ventilator for two and a half months and who "ultimately got better."

"Will you continue forever?" a woman intern asked.

"We go day by day. If he wants to go to three months, we'll probably go to three months," Luce said.

"What about insurance?"

"What about the cost to society?" the interns and residents asked.

The real issue was economic, Luce thought, but nobody, other than young doctors, ever talked about that. For a year, he and his colleagues had studied the withdrawal of life support from intensive care patients at the General and at another UCSF teaching facility, Moffitt Hospital. Funding or limited ICU beds was never given as the reason for withdrawing life support. Yet even if Mr. Davis survived this bout of PCP on the ventilator, he probably wouldn't live more than a month.

Ten years ago, intensive care units were full of hope. Physicians assumed that prolonging life was their duty (a relatively modern assumption) and they treated patients aggressively. When AIDS patients began coming, doctors pursued all possible therapies, even though some physicians thought it foolish to treat them in the expensive ICUs. By 1986, Luce and his colleagues had found that 87 percent of the PCP patients put on ventilators died at the General. At New York's Bellevue Hospital, the number dying in the hospital after being intubated on the ventilator reached 91 percent. Soon, fewer AIDS patients were requesting ventilators. More recently though, the survival rate at the General had jumped to 40 percent, although no one ever understood why. Other hospitals had found 50 to 58 percent survival rate following time spent on the ventilator. With the greater optimism, the advent of AZT and patients eager to aggressively attack the disease, by 1990 the General was seeing a fourfold increase in the number of PCP patients on ventilators. (The level has since declined as PCP has become less common.) Yet only one ventilator patient in any of the studies had lived more than a year after leaving the hospital.

Nobody addressed that issue. Doctors weren't allowed to talk about it because it was considered unseemly. Society wasn't interested in wrestling with it. And politicians, for the most part, kept their distance. People such as Mr. Davis, the elderly, or patients with massive head injuries might require major expenditures to keep them alive. Yet the problem was that society was spending millions of dollars on citizens who would never be productive again.

More and more doctors were confronting the principle of social justice. Limited medical resources were being parceled out. Every one of these patients was preventing women from getting maternity care, Luce thought. "All of us who are conscientious physicians are realizing somewhere in ourselves that a lot of the things we're doing ultimately mean that there's less money to spend on something else. It's all too abstract. Most people can't really grapple with it other than to say, 'Something is wrong here.'"

Luce told the house staff that if they believed it was an injustice to keep the patient on the ventilator so long, they would have to convince the patient and his family.

With his clean-cut good looks, sun-bleached hair, and red bow tie, John Luce resembles the Stanford English major he once was. His looks can deceive. Luce's political leanings are decidedly liberal. As a young politico, he worked for the California Democratic Party during the rise of its nemesis, Ronald Reagan. Back then, Luce earned a living as a medical writer doing articles for *Look* magazine, *Esquire* and *Rolling Stone*. He wrote a book with Dr. David Smith, about Smith's Haight Ashbury Free Medical Clinic, a place that offered care to drugged-out hippies and the poor. (Black-and-white photos of hippies from the Haight by photographer Irving Penn still share office wall space with crayoned drawings by Luce's kids.) Luce went to medical school in order to be a better science writer. He never returned to writing—except to write lucid articles in medical journals.

An idealist, he believed that one of the worst things to happen to medicine was the introduction of profit. Not surprisingly, he came to UC Med Center and the General where he specialized in pulmonary medicine and studied how to withdraw life support from patients.

When AIDS had come along, no lung specialist but Luce had been interested. In 1981, he saw the first patient with the mysterious new disease at the hospital. He'd been involved with AIDS before anyone knew it was an epidemic. Early on he told novelist Diane Johnson, the wife of a UC physician, that this disease was the most important medical story of the century, and it didn't yet have a name. He performed bronchoscopies on gay men with PCP before anyone knew AIDS was a communicable disease. Frequently doctors and nurses were splashed with the blood of patients with the mysterious disease. And sometimes patients' secretions splattered on their faces. For a year and a half, Luce and others who worked with him didn't take precautions against patients' body fluids.

Even after it was known that AIDS was a communicable disease and that health-care workers needed to protect themselves, Luce and other doctors and nurses still took risks. Once, while Luce was assisting in a bronchoscopy, an AIDS patient coughed blood in Luce's eye. "It was like being shot in the back," Luce recalled. He felt the depressed feeling "you feel when you're in danger." Stark. Horrid.

"Here I was looking at a patient." The one set of goggles in the room was worn by the doctor-in-training. The AIDS patient was bleeding. The doctor-in-training was in a semi-panic. Luce was there to try to help him stop the bleeding. "Part of me said, 'You are a doctor. You're job is to stop the bleeding.' And the other part of me said, 'Run out of this room as fast as you can to avoid shitting in your pants and to wash out your eyes.'

"The minute the coast was clear I ran across to the laboratory and flushed out my eyes, covered them with water and came back in the room." It was obvious to the patient that Luce had run out in panic.

Later that afternoon, Luce again washed out his eye. After discussing the situation with a number of his infectious-disease colleagues, he had his blood drawn to test for hepatitis exposure. The AIDS test didn't yet exist. And while waiting for the results, he was given the hepatitis vaccine, because he had not previously been immunized.

It marked the first time Luce looked death in the face. "Shit," he said, "there were no published risks yet from splashes. Everybody dealing with AIDS patients was coming to terms with the disease."

Since then, Luce has been more careful. He wears glasses now, primarily for protection. And he wears them all the time. He gowns and gloves, and when he draws blood from an AIDS patient, he does it with a calm hand. He sits down. He takes his time. "I think I know how to deal with it," he said, "and my fear has receded somewhat."

He's continued to work with AIDS patients. He's contributed to more than a dozen papers on AIDS and probably has collected every major article written about AIDS. "It's part of my life," he said. "I've never lost interest in it."

The comatose Mr. Davis remained oblivious to the controversy his status was creating. Eight more days had passed. On January 24, forty-one days after he had been put on the ventilator, the interns, the residents and Luce once again formed a circle in the hallway outside Mr. Davis's room. All the ICU beds were full. Pressure wasn't going to lessen any time soon. (That same week, the *Bay Area Reporter*, a San Francisco gay newspaper, printed its revised obituary policy: "Due to an unfortunately large number of obituaries," it read, the newspaper "must now restrict obits to 200 words.")

Mr. Davis was doing fine—for a man on a vent. One of the residents described his condition as "stone-cold stable."

Dr. Juliana Matthews, a onetime dancer with the Los Angeles Ballet, had tried to bring Mr. Davis up from his coma for a third time by reducing his intake of Valium and morphine. His eyes were tracking. He focused on the former ballerina with her perfect appearance and distant gaze. But his breathing was incredibly short. Like an octopus under attack, he fought the vent. When she asked him questions he nodded. He gave her the impression he wanted to remain on the ventilator.

"The only problem with that," she said to the circle of doctors, "is that he thinks it's December fourteenth and he's been here for one day."

If the patient was incapable of making the decision, then his family would have to make it for him. Mr. Davis's mother, a hard-working, deeply religious woman, had had no contact with her son in years, until they'd reconciled shortly before his hospitalization. From her home in Ohio, Mrs. Davis was trying to understand the problem. Nobody she knew in her small town had a gay son, an IV-drug-using son or a son with AIDS. She loved her boy and wanted to give God time to save him. She didn't want to be responsible for ending her child's life. That meant more time on the vent.

Luce asked about the possibility of the mother coming for a visit. She'd already come once, on a trip subsidized by her town. She couldn't take any additional time off from work.

Briefly, one resident considered giving the patient a paralytic agent while letting him be aware of what was going on.

"Too cruel," resident Matthews said. "That's too cruel." A general rule at the hospital was that if a patient was paralyzed he had also to be sedated.

"I don't think we want to wake him up and make him miserable just to tell him life is going to be miserable," Luce said, "unless we give him drugs to make him less miserable."

"At what point, John, do you say this is futility of care?" a female resident inquired.

He didn't have an answer.

It's very hard to die in an ICU. Only 25 percent of patients who die in ICUs do so despite care. The rest die because they've had support withdrawn. "It's unusual for these people to outfox us," Luce said, especially young men with strong hearts.

Much of the time, the physician felt he and the other doctors were stockbrokers for disease, giving a patient and his family advice. "Despite the fact that this hospital knows more about this disease than probably any hospital in the world," he said, "we still have a moving target. We still are constantly trying to educate ourselves and we still, despite our efforts, don't know, a good part of the time, what we're doing."

As chief of staff in 1989, and head of the executive committee, Luce dealt frequently with hospital policy on AIDS. The General provided an ongoing forum. "This is the place where things happen," Luce said. "This is the place where everything that is right or wrong about medicine comes to a head."

Regularly, resident Matthews was telephoning Mrs. Davis, trying to make her understand the futility of her son's situation. The mother told the resident about herself, about everyone she'd known who had died, including her husband and baby. When her son had contacted her for the first time in years, he said he wanted to leave the drug milieu and come home. She was praying for a miracle. In the meantime, the mother had joined a support group. In it, she met a mother from another town whose son had been on a ventilator for three months, had the support withdrawn, and died.

Mrs. Davis said she'd have to think about giving permission to take her son off the vent. She'd have to get used to the thought of her young son dying.

Luce had advised Matthews and the rest of the house staff that the final decision on Mr. Davis and on other intubated patients might rest with the United States Supreme Court. In the Nancy Cruzan case, then pending before the Court, a young woman had been comatose for seven years, following a car crash. If she continued to be tube fed, she might live another thirty years. The Missouri courts had held that her family did not have the right to stop medical care despite family members' contention that the woman would not have wanted to live that way. (In June 1990, the Supreme Court decided by five to four that a state could prevent a family from withdrawing life support from a comatose patient. The justices left it up to each state to determine the condition under which treatment could be stopped. In California, relatives are permitted to authorize removal of life support and tube feeding from the terminally ill.)

On one day when Matthews and the mother talked, the woman seemed reconciled to withdrawing support, but she was concerned that she didn't yet have enough money to bring her son's body back to Ohio.

"I need more time to get the money together," she said.

Matthews consulted an intensive-care-unit social worker, who advised her that the body could be kept in cold storage for a month. She relayed the information to the mother and she added, "It costs a lot to keep him on the ventilator." That was the only time costs were ever mentioned.

The mother agreed to let her son die.

For several days after the ventilator was withdrawn, Mr. Davis breathed on his own. On the 48th day of his hospitalization, his breathing was uncoordinated, his appearance agonal. The doctors stopped the antibiotics and the drawing of his blood. He died sixteen hours later. His medical bills came to over one hundred forty thousand dollars. They were paid by the city, state and federal governments.

To Kill a Drug

The discoverer of Q was still affable, still charming. But by the spring of 1990, the pressure on McGrath was palpable. At times he wondered what he'd done.

"I got thrown off a cliff," he said, "and haven't hit bottom yet. On the way down I'm bumping into things like rocks that happen to come from the side. There's no stopping it. The only thing that will stop it is when there's proof that it does or doesn't work. Until that happens, it's going to be rock and roll."

Although he'd done his best to hide his cooperation, when Project Inform's Martin Delaney had questions about Q, McGrath answered. He'd been in the eye of the storm and quietly, yet distinctly, he'd taken a stand. "I know if I were infected with HIV I would want to have access to everything that had some suggestion of activity," McGrath said. "I know that as a physician I'd be a lot more likely to get access than your random person. So at a very gut level, I can understand Martin's motivation and the entire [AIDS] community's motivation. I'm not against it. That's not to say I'm spitting in the faces of standard clinical trial testing. I'm not spitting in either face. I can understand the needs of both."

Delaney called him a hero: "He demonstrated he cares as much about the plight of patients as any patient activist we've ever met. He delivered on everything we've asked of him. That shouldn't be unusual. He only responded as a normal human being. It only showed us how abnormal so many other scientists have been. He's the first researcher who shared our frustration about unnecessary delays. He was not fettered by bullshit. He risked his career to deal with us."

That hadn't impressed the East Coast establishment, which was painting an image of McGrath as a scientific villain. A *New York Times* article that ran on September 19, 1989, on the first page of the Science Section was so critical of Q that according to McGrath, the story "made it poison." The article blamed the deaths of three men on the Project Inform Compound Q study. One had gone into a coma and recovered only to choke on vomit five days later and die. A second was said to have suffered paralysis, blindness and confusion after taking the Chinese Q. He recovered but died afterward. A third took it and, according to the article, committed suicide. A spokesman for ACT UP, a biomedical ethicist and others criticized the underground tests. Some called them shocking, chilling and unethical.

"Unlike federally approved studies," the article said, "the private study was not overseen by an impartial committee to look after the interests of desperate patients and to protect them from being harmed by the research . . ." The FDA, the article said, was conducting an investigation.

Shortly afterward, the FDA called on Project Inform to stop its unsanctioned drug trial. Q was doomed, or so it appeared.

The FDA checked into the accusations. The men who had died while taking the Chinese Q had been in the late stages of AIDS. The suicide patient had pulmonary Kaposi's sarcoma, a disease that kills quickly. When Q failed to help the KS, the man quit the painful lavage procedure that washed his lungs and extended life, and asked for a morphine drip to make his last days more comfortable. "He let nature take its course," Delaney said. The patient who suffered blindness and paralysis recovered and did a videotape describing his experience for future patients. Six weeks later, he suffered a neuropathy, a degeneration of the nervous system common to AIDS patients. "What he died of," Delaney said, "wasn't totally clear." The third patient had gone in and out of a coma, vomited in his sleep and acquired a fatal case of pneumonia.

Six months passed. The investigation over, the FDA made a shocking announcement. Project Inform was given authority to conduct an official GLQ223 trial. (Instead of smuggling Q from China, the group would acquire it from Genelabs, the American maker of Q.) Despite that, the attacks on Q continued.

"Taking the drug can be worse than taking nothing," said Harvard's Dr. Thomas Chalmers, associate director of the technology assessment group, in a front-page New York Times article. The piece indicated that Q was being tested on AIDS patients before it had proven to be effective in the test tube. Harvard's Dr. Jerome Groopman of the New England Deaconess Medical Center had tested Q in his lab, and, according to the Times, "had found the drug to be completely ineffective."

"One interpretation of this is that he's calling us guilty of scientific fraud," McGrath said coolly, "if you're paranoid and stuff like that." Only a few years before, Groopman and the General's Volberding had been the young turks of AIDS. By the late '80s and early '90s, they'd become the AIDS establishment and McGrath was the young rebel.

Groopman, McGrath complained, hadn't tried to replicate his Q experiments. The Harvard researcher had used plastic dishes to test infected macrophages. McGrath only used Teflon. A macrophage stuck to plastic responds differently than does a macrophage suspended in Teflon. The Teflon macrophage, McGrath contended, more closely resembled macrophage environment in the human body. McGrath felt "comforted that what we were measuring in our Teflon system duplicated what we saw in whole blood." He suggested that he and Groopman coauthor a paper on Q's varying response in vitro to plastic and Teflon. Instead, the response had come in the comments Groopman made to the New York Times.

Other labs had had difficulty with plastic dishes and Q, too. McGrath assigned his researcher, Isabelle Gaston, sometimes referred to as "Ms. Q," and other times as "Q-on-wheels," to teach various labs how to work with macrophages and Teflon. They were able to replicate the experiment.

In a formal complaint he filed with the dean of Harvard Medical School, Project Inform's Delaney charged that Groopman had intervened at the FDA to try to stop federal government from granting Project Inform permission to study Q. Another Harvard researcher,

Delaney charged, had contacted Sandoz, Genelabs' corporate partner, asking that the quarter-million-dollar grant be denied to the renegade group. In a written response, Harvard said that Groopman and others were only doing their duty as scientists and that it could find no evidence of wrongdoing.

Despite the public attacks, the FDA gave Project Inform authority to conduct the drug trial, and Sandoz came forward with the money.

At a night meeting held in the Women's Building (a gathering place for liberal causes) in the Mission District of San Francisco, Delaney stood before several hundred sad-faced men and recounted the data his study had collected. In addition to people with AIDS, the media and a few doctors from the General had come to listen. Researcher Gaston stood against a wall scribbling notes. Sometimes when Delaney spoke, his phraseology and the contents of his statement sounded so much like McGrath that chills ran through Gaston's body.

The reviews on Q were mixed but hopeful. Typically, patients complained of a week-long flu after infusion. Some found no benefit. For most, the early studies indicated moderate improvement. Delaney and the Project Inform doctors believed that if they could find the right dosage and give it at the right intervals, they might be able to extend life.

Q remained popular with the more adventurous HIV-positive free-lance drug shoppers. Buyers' clubs continued to purchase Q from China. Doctors in Los Angeles; New York; Washington, D.C.; St. Louis and Miami gave Q to patients requesting it. For those who couldn't afford doctors' fees, living-room clinics, with names such as CliniQ and Uncle Gene's Lab, offered bargain-rate infusions.

Isabelle Gaston's friend, Chris Adams, the gay writer, considered taking Q. He discussed it with Isabelle; if something happened to him while on it, he didn't want her to feel responsible. Chris joined the Genelabs Q drugs trials and began taking it at regular intervals.

Q came to be seen as a high-risk, possibly high-gain drug. Ever since the Project Inform study had determined that patients with fewer than 100 T cells should not take Q, there had been no further reports of comas or dementia. The absence of the terrible toxicity came as a tremendous relief to McGrath. "The last thing I want to do is be the father of a drug that knocks off a lot of people and then doesn't do anything," he said.

After several years with Q, McGrath had concluded that "it's remarkably easy to kill an AIDS drug. It just seems like anybody who develops an AIDS drug has more enemies than friends. It's in part because AIDS drug development is a multimillion-dollar business. Look at all the different companies. They're all backing their own horse. They're businesses. They have no interest in somebody else's drug doing anything. So automatically that puts you in the minority," McGrath said with his rat-tat-tat laugh. "I'm not a business and I'm still getting the flak." Rat-tat-tat.

"Any time you start challenging dogma, you get criticized by the ninety percent of the people who establish that dogma," he said. "That's been the story of my scientific career anyway."

He had no choice. Somewhere along the journey, McGrath realized that his research into Q and his involvement with the renegade Project Inform could derail his academic career. McGrath was cornering the market on AIDS lymphomas and operating the Q counter as well. Although not up for tenure, he'd been evaluated. The message carried a sting. His work was too diffuse and not thought to be significant. Even if Q possessed all the properties in vivo that it had in vitro, even if it helped save lives, McGrath felt it wouldn't help his standing at the university.

There were those who believed that McGrath's enthusiasm could be his undoing. At scientific meetings, when others gave crisp presentations, McGrath might pull up to the podium, remove his glasses and, some thought, "get a little wild."

For a moment he had been the media's darling, the golden boy of AIDS research. Now he went unnoticed by the public and tarred by fellow researchers. He was, as he said, able to take it.

The political naïf had taken a cram course in politics and human behavior. Q, he recognized, forever was entwined with radical politics. It had been used to change the machinery and a lot of scientists resented it. Many wanted to return to the good old days when placebo control trials were the norm. "I think the AIDS community has made their wishes known," McGrath said, "and that is that they have access to drugs. History will judge if that is the right thing to do or not. Fortunately or unfortunately, Q was the drug they picked to do it."

Long after Project Inform had disclosed its preliminary findings to the public, a paper detailing the research was accepted by the journal *AIDS*. It would run in the same issue as the paper describing the General's early GLQ223 trials, written by Dr. James Kahn. Project Inform held a small victory party for its leadership at Victor's Restaurant in the elegant old St. Francis Hotel. McGrath joined the celebrants.

At the Sixth International Conference on AIDS held in San Francisco in June of 1990, Delaney and AIDS doctor Larry Waites disclosed the results of their research. Of forty-six patients infused with Q on a monthly basis while continuing to take AZT, eight men with T cell counts between 100 and 200 had, after five months, normal T cell counts of around 1,000. About half the other patients increased their T cell count but the numbers remained dangerously low. A quarter of the patients showed no improvement.

For disclosing information before it was published, Delaney was publicly attacked at the conference by then editor of the *New England Journal of Medicine*, Dr. Arnold Relman, who called him "irresponsible," and his findings "black magic." "Everybody wants to see a safe and effective treatment for AIDS," Relman said, "but we don't want to see people using an undocumented, untested drug that could kill."

The General's preliminary findings demonstrated no lasting benefit in patients given Q and a toxicity in those who were neurologically impaired. But Dr. Kahn, investigator for the trial, pointed out that his original method of treatment, using one fast infusion, appeared not to be effective. In later work, he did what Project Inform had done, and gave slow-drip infusions at regular intervals.

The rift between the hospital and Delaney had begun to heal. Volberding and Delaney once again were saying pleasant things about one another. Kahn offered congratulatory words to Delaney at the AIDS conference. And to reporters, Kahn said he thought nothing could stop the development of Q now. "Not that it's so important necessarily, but there is so much attention on it. If it's effective, we need to get the word out. And if it's toxic, we need to get the word out."

McGrath remained hopeful. Both the General and Project Inform continued to conduct Phase I trials to determine the safety of Q.

"Normally, if you're working on something that's unpopular or you can't get it funded, then maybe you shouldn't work on it anymore. Then the heat lets up because you're no longer working on something that's unpopular," McGrath said.

"Q won't let up. I can't let up. I can't jump off. It's got to be taken to its logical end. Either it has activity or it doesn't and we're going to take all kinds of flak for political and scientific reasons, and that's just part of the game. The only issue will be whether it works in people."

Where to Draw the Line

This is a little complicated," said professor Molly Cooke to her ethics class, "but this is real life, folks." An internist at the General and associate professor of clinical medicine at UCSF, Cooke told the medical students about a dilemma she'd faced in clinic the previous week. Her female patient had been nervous about contracting AIDS. When her wayward husband wanted to come home after a sojourn of crack and sex, the patient had insisted he be tested for the AIDS virus. His results came back positive. Now, Cooke told the eager medical students, "He knows and she knows.

"The person who doesn't know," Cooke said, was the other woman whom he had seen during the separation and whom, the doctor suspected, he was continuing to see.

Cooke's patient often sees the other woman. It would be fairly easy for the physician to find out the other woman's name.

"What do people think about my obligation?"

It's vintage Cooke.

232

The things that trouble her, the issues to which she devotes herself, are the in-between issues. "If it were clear what to do," she says, prowling the front of the room with the grace of a Siamese cat, "everyone would have done it."

Sometimes, when TV crews come to do AIDS stories at the General, they interview Cooke but then don't use what she says because she doesn't deal in ten-second snippets. She's too cerebral. If she hadn't gone into medicine, Cooke might have remained with her love of literature, becoming a poet or a novelist.

At thirty-eight, Cooke serves as a role model for a younger generation of women physicians. From the time she was chief resident in medicine in 1980–81, Cooke has dealt with AIDS. Married to Dr. Volberding, head of AIDS at the General, they have three young children. When they were very little, Cooke sometimes brought her babies to work in a basket. Even now, when daycare fails, she brings her youngest to class.

She tells the class her patient had tried to warn the other woman, dropping broad hints like, "'If I slept with people who did crack, I'd get HIV tested.' The other woman wasn't hearing. So do I have an obligation? This is not just anybody. This is an identified individual."

A red-haired medical student was the first to react: "You have an obligation if you know her name."

"I don't know her name," Cooke said. "My patient knows her name."

Another, older female student in a ponytail suggested "a diminishing chain of responsibility." The man has the greatest responsibility, then his wife, and least of all the physician. To her, a doctor is no different from anyone else.

Only recently had the medical community recognized the importance of a patient learning his HIV status early. That recognition came with availability of AZT, the only drug that had been proven to extend an AIDS patient's life. What's stated less often is the importance of notifying a patient so that he can alter his behavior to avoid transmitting the disease.

"This is a very difficult situation," Cooke told the students at UC Medical Center. "Do I have an obligation to compensate for everybody else along the line?"

"It's not really your business," another student interjected, "because the only way you know is that your patient told you about someone else. It's almost an invasion of his privacy."

Most of Cooke's clinic cases she's forgotten by the time she arrives home to feed the kids. This one gnawed at her.

She sat on a table in front of the classroom, her lanky arms reaching out as if she were pulling answers out of the minds of her students. A child of the '60s, she was wearing an unassuming antique rose jersey and charcoal cords. Her wavy blond hair hung loose. Pretty and thin, she could have been one of those natural-looking models for the Tweeds catalogue. But for the puffiness under her eyes, the badge of the working mother, she could pass for twenty-eight.

"I made no effort in the course of this discussion to find out who this person was," she said. "If I knew the person's name I would feel more responsible."

She had met the husband when his wife, her patient, had been hospitalized. A man of street charm, the husband seemed to her to be approachable. She asked her patient if the husband would come to the clinic for a talk. Cooke didn't think he would ever be willing to tell the other woman, "but he could give me permission to talk with this other woman."

Cooke hopped off the table and walked as she analyzed. Two principles were in conflict. Doctors, she said, have a special responsibility toward their doctor-patient relationship. They also have a public-health responsibility, she said, which is much less intense.

Someone asked if she was saying, "I care less about this person who I don't know because I don't know her. It's less important to me that she might have HIV because I don't know her"?

Cooke agreed. "There are a lot of people getting infected out there. I wish none of them got infected. I can't intervene with everybody. Where do I draw the line?"

"Where you can't do it," a still idealistic student replied.

Nobody said it, but they were talking about one person sentencing another to death and a physician's obligation to try to prevent it.

A Syrian student had a different perspective. "I don't see any good that could happen from not revealing the truth. Forgetting about all the legal things, even forgetting about one's profession, being a doctor, just being a person. . . . The woman should be told. I'm very surprised that her friend wouldn't have told her by now."

"What about for me?" Cooke pressed.

"I don't see the point of not telling her. Then again, my background is not from so individualistic a society. Therefore, I could not probably see some of the advantages of being so individual. For me, I find it very, very, very intuitive. I would pick up the phone and tell her right now."

"There's only a limited amount of time I have and I have to decide what to do with it," Cooke responded. "I recognize that in fact as this situation is playing itself out, this woman may never get told and may become HIV infected."

The Syrian pursued his line of reasoning. "Maybe she already has it and she's also having intercourse with other people."

Cooke agreed: "There's a lot of bad things that can happen."

For years, Cooke had treated AIDS patients and studied the fear the virus arouses in physicians. Her interest grew out of her experience. She'd just given birth to their first child, when her husband began working at the General. While she was home on maternity leave, he saw the first Kaposi's sarcoma patient at the hospital. Then he saw a few Pneumocystis patients.

When Cooke returned from maternity leave, she took her team of doctors by to see the patients with the strange ailments, saying, "You're never going to see another case of this. This is a very rare tumor."

That fall (1981) it became obvious to Volberding, an oncologist by training, that the same people that were getting Pneumocystis were getting KS. You didn't have to be an epidemiologist to conclude that there was some common underlying problem.

Cooke remembered her husband saying, "There's something wrong with these people that's transmitted like an infectious disease that leads to the Pneumocystis and the KS.'" There were a lot of people coming to the same conclusion at the same time. About six weeks later, he told her, "It's transmitted like hepatitis B." (Hepatitis B is another blood-borne virus and is also an occupational hazard for health-care workers.)

She'd gone into medicine with a sense of invincibility. Suddenly she was considering personal risk. She wasn't sure what her duties were. The outdated Hippocratic Oath was no longer given to young doctors because, among other issues, it forbade surgery and abortions.

Early on, the hospital mounted an AIDS education program for its nurses and doctors. It worked, although by 1985 four nurses had quit the hospital when the administration refused to let them wear masks and gloves to bathe or medicate AIDS patients.

Cooke contended that the controversy led by Dr. Day, head of the hospital's orthopedic surgery, was another case of acknowledging fears.

"For years [the surgeons] have been saying 'AIDS is another reason why I'm glad I'm not an internist.' Then suddenly, they say, 'My God. These patients are coming to us, too.' "

Cooke recognized that surgeons are at greater risk. "You'd have to be crazy to contend that point." But she thought more was involved. AIDS was a hideous disease. Physicians as a group tended to have more anxiety over death than did the general public. Surgeons love to cure things, yet AIDS can't be cured. Based on her own surveys, Cooke argued that anxiety over a patient's homosexuality heightened the fear of AIDS among male physicians.

Often, the discussion at the General had deteriorated to the level of an internist telling a surgeon, "You have to operate on my patient." And the surgeon replying, "I'm not going to have an internist tell me what I have to do."

"There have been turf fights since time began," Cooke said. "We have never as a medical staff tried to deal with issues anywhere near this moral magnitude . . . This is quite a profound area that we're struggling with."

The ethics class she was teaching had been organized at the request of the medical students. Cooke had a longstanding interest in medical ethics and students' attitudes toward AIDS.

In a study she conducted of more than a thousand internal-medicine students at forty-one medical schools in the United States, Cooke found 66 percent fearful of contracting AIDS on the job; 10 percent had been stuck by a needle containing blood from a patient they believed to be HIV positive. One-fourth of those surveyed chose their training to avoid having to work with AIDS patients. A fourth also said they would look for work in areas where AIDS was not prevalent. More than a third said they would not accommodate HIV patients in their practice. Some 64 percent said they would accommodate AIDS patients. Cooke was concerned that there might not be enough physicians to care for future AIDS patients.

Her study emphasized the dichotomy between what the public expects of physicians and what physicians expect of themselves. "It may never have been true that physicians have been motivated as a profession by service to the extent that nurses are," Cooke said. "I think we share with the lay public some of these glorified ideals. When the profession is stressed, you start seeing some cracks."

As she traveled around the country, talking about ethics and anxiety, Cooke found predictable waves of fear in one hospital after another. The General had just gone through it before many others.

"There's a limit to how long you can go on being horribly anxious every day," she said. "Then you either say 'I can't tolerate this' or you do something internally that makes you less anxious, maybe a new way of understanding what your risk is or developing some kind of stoicism—line-of-duty stuff."

Cooke was on maternity leave with her third child, Emily, when the hospital announced the seroconversion of Jane Doe. The physician's reaction was very matter of fact: "Gee," she said, "we've had about seven hundred needle-sticks here, so I guess you'd expect us to have a seroconversion." People were shocked by what she said. In retrospect, Cooke recognizes, "It was an insensitive thing to say. . . . One way to interpret it is to say I was intellectualizing."

"When you're most aware of denial," Cooke observed, "is when it doesn't work. . . . Jane Doe made denial no longer work for people for whom it had worked until the fall of 1987."

Since then, Cooke has learned to deal with her fears. She believed that the risk was within the range that was expected of a physician. She weighed the alternatives. Her patients needed care. "If I'm not going to take care of them, then there are two options: One is that no one will take care of them. That definitely doesn't feel right. Or someone else will take care of them. Why should that someone else do it more than me?"

One Thread

$\bigwedge$ cop in a black-and-white patrol car kept watch, just in case. The First Annual International Conference on Jewish Medical Ethics held in January 1990 was supposed to be an intellectual exercise in ethics, not the sort of conference to draw a protest. Then Dr. Lorraine Day was invited.

The bristly, iconoclastic Rabbi Pinchas Lipner, dean of the Institute for Jewish Medical Ethics, had earlier received calls from physicians warning that Day was a fascist, a Nazi, a crazy and an hysteric. They accused her of lacing her speeches with scare tactics and of loosely doling out misinformation. Bay Area Physicians for Human Rights wrote Rabbi Lipner advising him to cancel Day's speech. They mailed copies of their letter to Jews in high places in the United States, England and Israel, pressure tactics that infuriated the rabbi but failed to dissuade him. He'd stood up to threats before. Shortly after the Israeli invasion of Lebanon, the rabbi had invited then Israeli defense minister Ariel Sharon to speak at the San Francisco Hilton Hotel. Protesters

238

threatened to blow up the hotel. Hundreds of picketers demonstrated. Still, Sharon spoke. So when doctors tried to convince the rabbi to uninvite Day, they were, he said, "talking to the wrong person." An Orthodox Jew in a city of very liberal ones, the rabbi had felt victimized for years by what he called Jewish McCarthyism. Now, he said, he saw it coming back to plague Day.

Michelle Roland, one of the Bay Area's most outspoken members of ACT UP, wrote the rabbi asking him to reconsider. The daughter of Jewish Berkeley activists, Roland was a first-year medical student at the University of California at Davis. In earlier skirmishes at the General and with federal AIDS officials, she'd proven to be unintimidated by authority. "Dr. Day's beliefs about HIV transmission have been discredited by all the leading authorities on HIV," she wrote. "Her fears are exactly that—fears. . . . The public is afraid of HIV. That fear becomes displaced onto people with HIV infection." She warned the rabbi that he would hear more from ACT UP.

Gary Carr, the head nurse practitioner at Ward 86, complained about Day in letters to the *Northern California Jewish Bulletin* and the *Bay Area Reporter*. He called the invitation "insulting." Although both he and the surgeon worked at the same hospital and both were focused on AIDS, the two had never met. But Carr knew what Day said and what she stood for, and he hated her views and the fact that she came from the same caring institution for which he worked. Carr's work resembles a messianic duty. "Her views on this subject," he wrote, "are well known to us and generally considered, at best, ridiculous and embarrassing and, at worst, part of a sinister political agenda."

Nevertheless, the invitation stood and Day accepted. Knowing the opposition to her presence, Rabbi Lipner reminded his audience that Jews have always defended freedom of speech. While the audience might not agree with Day's views, he pointed out, he supported her right to raise the issues "without intimidation or political pressure."

Some four hundred participants from across the world lunched on beer, kosher hot dogs and slaw. Only peanuts and football were missing. Although it was Super Bowl Sunday, the gymnasium at the imposing Herbrew Academy was full of somber-looking physicians seated on folding metal chairs. "Not a lot of sports fans here," a neurologist observed. Newspapers and TV would describe the frenzy after the game, but at the conference, it was two hours and ten minutes into the Super Bowl before Dr. Mervyn Silverman, the former head of San Francisco's health department and current president of the American Foundation for AIDS Research (AmFAR), asked if anyone knew the score.

In a cloud of gray men, long beards, and drab suits, Day stood out like an exclamation point. In her red-white-and-blue outfit, she was by far the most stylish figure in the room. What she said, however, made even more of an impression.

So many people were so suspicious of Day's motives that she began her speech with a disclaimer: "I have no political affiliations. I have no religious affiliations."

Her tone was melodic but her message cut. "When the United States decided to start a space program and they decided to train astronauts, which are about as expensive to train as physicians, they knew upon reentry of the space capsule that there would be tremendous heat. And if they didn't have special heat-shielding tiles, they would stand a chance of melting the entire space capsule and all those in it upon reentry. Did they say to the astronauts, 'Well, we haven't developed any heat-shielding material. We just suggest that you're astronauts and you're supposed to be tough. You can't have a risk-free environment. You just get in there; we'll see how it goes when you come back in.' They didn't do that. They said, 'Heat-shielding tiles will protect you as much as possible. And then you will have to take additional risks.'

"I have never suggested AIDS patients not be cared for. What I'm asking for is a reasonable amount of safety," she said. "I know of no AIDS research dollars that are going into any protective clothing or equipment for health-care workers," she said. Latex gloves that allow physicians to feel when they operate but are not penetrable by a needle or a sharp instrument would, she said, reduce the risk by 90 percent.

As Day spoke, a man of about forty, with slicked-back brown hair, wearing gold wire-rim glasses, a brown suit and carrying a worn leather briefcase quietly entered the room. He stood against a side wall, looking somewhat out of place and time. Impassively, Dr. Bill Schecter listened to Day, whose words he'd countered so many times before. Both frequently expressed fear for themselves. Both resented having been told early on that health-care workers were not at risk for AIDS. But while Day found the threat too great to allow her to continue operating at the General, Schecter arrived at another decision.

"This is a spine, open," Day was saying, exhibiting a gory color slide of blood, muscle and bone on the wall. "Those wires have to go into the spinal canal. How do I protect your spinal canal when I'm operating on you? I put my gloved finger in there to gently press the spinal cord out of the way while I put the wire through. I can't use an instrument on your spinal cord because I [risk] damage and may make you a paraplegic. . . . Where does the wire go? It goes into my finger. I will injure myself in this operation maybe four or five times during this procedure . . ."

On the wall, her slides projected more scenes from bloody operating rooms. "You need to have a good idea of what we do and why I'm talking about it the way I am. This is a drill. This is how the floor looks. Blood all over the place. This is how the linens look. Blood all over our feet. When we were told it wasn't dangerous to have it on our skin we had blood all over our legs. It would go through our gowns. We would almost always go home from the operating room with blood on our underwear because it soaked through our gowns. We were told that this is not dangerous. It turns out that it definitely is dangerous."

She zapped a picture of a physician on the wall. "All that blood that's on the face shield used to be on our faces. . . . This is what happens to us. It's not like watching Ben Casey on television and having a very clean field and no blood flying around."

In orthopedic surgery, she reminded the audience, "We drill and ream on bone. The bone is submerged in blood," she said, lurching into a typical Day analogy: "How would you like it if this weekend you decided to build a bookcase and you had power tools, power saws and power drills. But before you were allowed to build a bookcase I came over to your house and said, 'All right, before you are allowed to build this bookcase, I am going to submerge all your lumber in a vat of HIV-positive blood. Then start your power saws.'"

Her audience was still listening. No one walked out or shouted her down. And the police, finding no demonstrators, left in their squad car.

She questioned whether AIDS could be transmitted through French kissing, saliva, tears or urine. She castigated the CDC for not investigating and for misleading health-care workers.

Brothels in Reno must inform customers if a woman is HIV positive, Day observed, but patients don't have to tell their doctors.

"It's clear to me now and two years ago," Day concluded, "that we as health-care workers are not being told the whole truth and the public hasn't been either. . . . Why not take care of health-care workers who are taking care of AIDS patients?"

Day could not have anticipated her audience's reaction. The doctors applauded long and hard. A few even gave her a standing ovation.

Rabbi J. David Bleich, Ph.D., professor of Jewish law and ethics at Yeshiva University's Benjamin N. Cardozo School of Law rose to give the Jewish perspective.

His black yarmulke slung back on his head, he talked about a physician's responsibility to care for AIDS patients. "Physicians," he said, "have no greater responsibility than anyone else. . . . No individual is obligated to place himself in danger. He may if he chooses to do so. But he has no obligation to do so." Society, he said, has such an obligation. An individual, he asserted, does not. In a high-pitched voice, he said physicians have an obligation to preserve their own lives just as a mother sometimes must sacrifice her fetus to save her own life.

When he finished, Day and the audience clapped. Schecter remained impassive.

The panel discussion that followed was held on stage. Experts were seated at a long table drapped in a white cloth. Day sat isolated at one end. Dr. Silverman had scrunched his folding chair as close as he could to Schecter's, allowing maximum space between himself and Day. In a recent newspaper story he had referred to her as "Sweet Lorraine."

In front of the group, Silverman talked about the views that he and "Lorraine share." When she talked about him, she steadfastly called him "Dr. Silverman." He told the doctors that much is known about AIDS but that to alert the public to a rare possible transmission through a child's biting his sibling would "distort and confuse." His remarks were just the kind that Day would attack. The audience remained with her.

Occasionally Silverman was eloquent. He likened doctors to firemen and policemen. "We in the health-care profession have a monopoly and since we have a monopoly, I think we have an obligation to care."

The AIDS quilt, he said, has panels three feet by six feet, the approximate size of a casket. "Every one of them," he reminded his audience, "is somebody's child."

When it was Schecter's turn he thanked the group for allowing him to speak at "this very important panel." In a low voice, he introduced himself as "a surgeon in the civilian combat zone at San Francisco General Hospital."

"I see about a hundred people in clinic each Monday afternoon. I don't have time to provide pre- and postop [AIDS] testing and counseling. I personally think that is foolish. I treat every person as if they are infectious," he said.

Opposed to mandatory AIDS tests, he said, "The concept of the individual liberty to me is central. If you say we'll sacrifice individuality for the greater good, that to me is like pulling thread from my suit. Many times I have pulled one thread of my suit and just one thread has come out. But sometimes the whole seam opens up and the suit falls apart."

He said he believed that physicians who want mandatory testing "are really trying to figure out a way they can personally avoid operating on patients."

He told his audience about the operation he and other surgeons at the General had performed on the HIV-positive little boy brought from the Soviet Union. "Which brings us to the question is it okay for us to say to sick people, whether a five-and-a-half-year-old child or forty-five-year-old homosexual, is it okay to say that we're not going to take care of you?

"I'm not a Torah scholar," he said, sounding more rabbinical than the rabbi. "I approach this problem from the point of view of Leviticus," repeating the simple quote that guided his career: "'Neither shalt thou stand idly by the blood of thy neighbor.' That goes for all of us, whether we're professionals or not. It's particularly important for those who have education, training and experience to actually [be able to] do something about it.

"I operate on HIV-infected patients four days out of seven. Every morning when I'm shaving I think of what Maimonides said seven hundred years ago in his prayer for the physician: 'Preserve my strength that I may be able to restore strength of the rich and the poor, the good and the bad, the friend and the foe and,' dare I add, the heterosexual and the homosexual . . . 'let me see in the sufferer the man alone.'"

Applause was brief. "He's a very nice man," Rabbi Lipner said later, "but when it comes to Jewish law, he's an ignoramus." It wasn't that he misquoted, the Rabbi said, so much as it was that he "misinterpreted." "If I asked him to translate the Talmud, I don't think he could do sixth-grade work." Lipner seemed not to know that Schecter speaks and reads Hebrew fluently and frequently goes to Israel to teach medical classes to physicians—in Hebrew.

When it was over, Day was encircled by admirers questioning her, praising her and picking up her information sheets. It looked like she was offering free lottery tickets. Patiently Day conversed, giving time to her many allies.

For two hours following her speech Day remained seated onstage, answering questions, discussing the issues. The thirst for her information was enormous. Although the conference also featured pioneer heart surgeon Dr. Norman Shumway and Dr. Michael Bishop, the 1989 winner of the Nobel Prize in medicine, Day clearly was the star.

When the physicians filed back into the room for their dinner at seven thirty, Day was still at the panel table, answering questions. As she stood to leave, the crowd rose and gave her a standing ovation.

Two and a half hours before that, the physicians, anxious to reach Day, were lined up on the steps and clustered in the front of the room. Clutching his briefcase, Schecter brushed by. One couple approached to shake his hand. Then he passed unnoticed through the chaos and the excitement of the moment.

Postscript

Dr. Paul Volberding, one of the leading AIDS doctors in the nation, just completed his term as president of the International AIDS Society. He now spends much of his time away from the General shuttling to Washington, D.C., where he is involved in planning AIDS policy on research and drug development for the nation. He no longer sees many patients. Volberding worries that while the epidemic spreads—affecting patients "from ever more disadvantaged backgrounds"—the public is losing interest in the disease. At the General, he's concerned about the lack of space for AIDS care. With cramped quarters and additional patients, Volberding worries that the hospital could become a place in which tuberculosis, which is highly transmissible to HIV-infected people, could be spread from patient to patient in the waiting room, as well as to staff, many of whom are HIV positive.

Dr. Molly Cooke, Volberding's wife, now teaches introduction to clinical medicine to first- and second-year medical students at UCSF.

She continues to do research on AIDS ethics and works half a day a week in Ward 86.

Dr. Lorraine Day resigned from UCSF, divorced her surgeon husband and married a southern California attorney who had known her as a child and had seen her on *60 Minutes*. She moved to the Palm Springs area and, with the help of her husband, published a book, *AIDS: What the Government Isn't Telling You*, which has sold well. Paul Harvey recommended it as must reading on his daily radio show. Day has also started Americans for Common Sense, an organization dedicated to getting "the AIDS epidemic under control." In her letter to potential members she writes, "We have had enough of the incompetent approach taken by the government, by organized medicine and by the gay activists." Her group will push for widespread AIDS testing, funds for research into "all methods of transmission of AIDS," telling adolescents that condoms do not provide safe sex and, once someone is diagnosed, informing that person's sexual contacts.

Some observers contend that when Day left the hospital, she lost her primary platform and her heavyweight impact on the national debate. But she's still effective among her surgical colleagues. In 1992, the American Academy of Orthopedic Surgeons overwhelmingly endorsed a move to have surgeons tested for AIDS and a restriction of privileges for those who test positive. Day led the discussion in favor of the policy. "It was," she said, "the only responsible medical organization that did that."

Dr. Bill Schecter continues to operate on patients regardless of their HIV status. Long after Day left for the lecture circuit, Schecter continued to put on his protective gear and perform surgery four days out of seven. He's never worn the space suit. Recently, San Francisco General began using safer, costlier needles and syringes. And health-care workers performing blood-splattering procedures now protect themselves with clear plastic face shields.

Dr. Michael McGrath still does research on GLQ223. The drug is in its second (efficacy) phase of a three-part drug trial. Project Inform remained optimistic about Q. But in the gay underground, once so enamored of the Chinese medicine, Q no longer is the drug of choice.

People have moved on to other treatments. "When all is said and done," McGrath recently said, "I think it's going to be a good drug."

Vince DeGenova, the nurse in charge of selecting subjects for Q and other drug trials at the General, left his job last year when he became ill with AIDS. At home, he either sleeps or tries to forget. "Continue telling the story," he advised. "Plant a tree. . . . lie under it and remember that there go I but for the grace of God."

Teddy, the younger of the two men infused with GLQ223 in the General's drug trials, felt his health deteriorate after he was taken off Q following his participation in the trials. He became increasingly ill, quit seeing many of his friends or even talking on the phone. He died in late May 1992. Harold, the patient with whom he shared a hospital room, could not be found.

J.B. Molaghan and Gary Carr still run Ward 86. Last year, the number of patients coming to Ward 86 increased by 30 percent while there was no increase in staff. Under the pressure, the uniqueness of the unit was beginning to fade. To some, it felt more like a typical county clinic. "Every time there's a turn in AIDS," Carr said, "it's a turn for the worse."

Mary Rathbun, the cookie lady of Ward 86, a.k.a. Brownie Mary, was still volunteering at the General with her chocolate-chocolate chip cookies and her peanut-butter-chip cookies. In July 1992, Mary was arrested for possession with intent to sell marijuana in a raid by the Drug Enforcement Administration. She was in the middle of baking twenty dozen marijuana brownies—eighteen dozen for the AIDS patients she called "my kids," two for her personal use. Marijuana can ease pain and nausea and stimulate the appetite of AIDS patients with "wasting syndrome." When she was arrested in the early '80s, Mary was engaged in a for-profit "cottage industry." This time, however, her brownies were free, and she offered free delivery. Although she was released on five thousand dollars bail, Mary was weepy and upset. But she said she was willing to go to jail for her principles. She became a San Francisco heroine. August 25, 1992, was named Mary Rathbun Day. At the time of her arrest, she was seventy years old.

Dr. John Luce, the former chief of staff, is now medical director of quality assurance for the hospital. Since Lorraine Day left, he no longer hears complaints from patients or their lovers about surgical care. He still sees AIDS patients in the intensive care unit.

Dr. Eric Goosby, an AIDS doctor who saw patients in the methadone clinic, now administers the Ryan White Title I and Title II programs for the Health Resources and Services Administration in Rockville, Maryland. The federal program disburses over two million dollars for AIDS care to cities and states each year.

Dr. Gerald Hill, the American Indian doctor in the General's emergency room, is now the director of the Center of American Indian and Minority Health at the University of Minnesota Duluth Medical School. The center recruits and trains American Indian medical students. Periodically Hill returns to San Francisco and works in the General's ER.

Melissa Bartick graduated from UCSF Medical School and began her internship in Cambridge, Massachusetts. She had planned to specialize in pediatrics but switched to internal medicine where she could treat the people she called "the disenfranchised."

Jane Doe just turned thirty. She continues to work at San Francisco General, where few people know her identity. Her feistiness remains intact. She called a friend to express her outrage: "Isn't this scandalous? Isn't this horrible? Can you believe this?" she said to the answering machine. A few weeks later, she called, once again reaching the machine. She left this message: "It's still scandalous! I'll keep you posted."

Although her T cells have dropped, Jane Doe feels well and has taken up ethnic dancing.

She is no longer alone. A second San Francisco General nurse learned she was HIV positive from an apparent on-the-job accident. (Nationwide, the CDC reports thirty-one documented cases of health-care workers who have acquired HIV from on-the-job accidents. The CDC lists sixty-five others as "possible" cases. The real figures are believed to be much higher.) The nurse discovered her status after taking a blood test for a life insurance policy. She believes she contracted the disease in 1983, when she cut herself while caring for an AIDS patient in an intensive care unit at the General.

The Centers for Disease Control estimates that one million Americans are HIV positive. By the year 2000, a projected 30 to 110 million people will be infected with the AIDS virus worldwide.

Index